Atlas of Orbital Tumors

December 18, 1999

To Marlon Maus —
We really enjoy or friendship
and academic association —
We hope you enjoy the books

Best regards,

Jerry Shields
Carol Shields

Atlas of Orbital Tumors

Jerry A. Shields, M.D.

Director, Ocular Oncology Service
Wills Eye Hospital
Professor of Ophthalmology
Thomas Jefferson University
Philadelphia, Pennsylvania

Carol L. Shields, M.D.

Surgeon, Ocular Oncology Service
Wills Eye Hospital
Associate Professor of Ophthalmology
Thomas Jefferson University
Philadelphia, Pennsylvania

LIPPINCOTT WILLIAMS & WILKINS
A **Wolters Kluwer** Company
Philadelphia • Baltimore • New York • London
Buenos Aires • Hong Kong • Sydney • Tokyo

Acquisitions Editor: Christine Battle Rullo/Paula Callaghan
Developmental Editor: Delois Patterson
Manufacturing Manager: Dennis Teston
Production Manager: Jodi Borgenicht
Production Editor: Jonathan Geffner
Cover Designer: QT Graphics
Indexer: Nancy Newman
Compositor: Lippincott Williams & Wilkins Desktop Division

Printed and bound in China

9 8 7 6 5 4 3 2 1

Library of Congress Cataloging-in-Publication Data
Shields, Jerry A.
    Atlas of orbital tumors / Jerry A. Shields, Carol L. Shields.
        p.   cm.
    Includes bibliographical references and index.
    ISBN 0-7817-1917-8
        1. Eye-sockets—Tumors—Atlases.   I. Shields, Carol L.   II. Title.
    RC280.E9 S548   1999
    616.99′284–dc21

                                                                98-39677
                                                                CIP

Care has been taken to confirm the accuracy of the information presented and to describe generally accepted practices. However, the authors and publisher are not responsible for errors or omissions or for any consequences from application of the information in this book and make no warranty, expressed or implied, with respect to the contents of the publication.

The authors and publisher have exerted every effort to ensure that drug selection and dosage set forth in this text are in accordance with current recommendations and practice at the time of publication. However, in view of ongoing research, changes in government regulations, and the constant flow of information relating to drug therapy and drug reactions, the reader is urged to check the package insert for each drug for any change in indications and dosage and for added warnings and precautions. This is particularly important when the recommended agent is a new or infrequently employed drug.

Some drugs and medical devices presented in this publication have Food and Drug Administration (FDA) clearance for limited use in restricted research settings. It is the responsibility of the health care provider to ascertain the FDA status of each drug or device planned for use in their clinical practice.

To our six wonderful children
Jerry, Patrick, Billy Bob, Maggie Mae, John, and Charlotte Nelle,
who have provided us with endless hours of entertainment
during the preparation of this book.

Contents

Foreword

Atlas of Orbital Tumors has a pleasing format and contains myriad pearls of clinical information. It has been carefully assembled, with an elegant balance of clinical, pathologic, and diagnostic photographs and illustrations. Because of it, clinicians will make more frequently correct diagnoses of comparatively rare orbital tumors and simulating inflammatory pseudotumors. It will be, and deserves to be, a major resource for those in training as well as for highly specialized orbitologists.

Carol and Jerry Shields are good personal and professional friends and are among a select group of the most phenomenal husband and wife ophthalmic teams that has ever existed. Spanning intraocular and adnexal tumors, their combined ophthalmic oncology practice and experience are indisputably the most extensive in the world today and serve as the basis for the development of this atlas. They publish prolifically, travel widely, organize symposia and courses, and yet are able to maintian a rich and admirable family life, which includes six wonderful children.

Atlas of Orbital Tumors is yet another ornament in their scintillating careers and a gift to ophthalmology.

Frederick A. Jackobiec, M.D., D.Sc.
Henry Willard Williams Professor of Ophthalmology
Professor of Pathology
Chairman, Department of Ophthalmology
Harvard Medical School, and
Chief of Ophthalmology
The Massachusetts Eye and Ear Infirmary
Boston, Massachusetts

Preface

For about 25 years, we have a pursued a full-time medical and surgical practice of ophthalmic oncology at Wills Eye Hospital of Thomas Jefferson University in Philadelphia. During that time, we have enjoyed the unusual opportunity to document the clinical and histopathologic characteristics of most neoplasms and related conditions that occur in the eyelids, conjunctiva, intraocular structures, and orbit. In addition, we have been able to photographically document our extensive experience in the clinical diagnosis and management of these conditions. We have incorporated this material into comprehensive lectures on ocular tumors and pseudotumors that we frequently share with ophthalmologists and other physicians. A number of clinicians and ophthalmic pathologists have encouraged us to assemble our excellent slide collection into comprehensive color atlases to assist physicians with recognition of the various ocular tumors and related conditions. Consequently, we have produced three volumes, entitled *Atlas of Eyelid and Conjunctival Tumors*, *Atlas of Intraocular Tumors*, and *Atlas of Orbital Tumors*.

This particular atlas covers tumors and pseudotumors that affect the orbit. Some of these conditions are common and relatively harmless and require no treatment. Some benign lesions are not a threat to the patient's systemic health but can cause serious visual impairment and cosmetic deformity. Some malignant tumors may pose a threat to the patient's vision and life. Imaging studies like computed tomography and magnetic resonance imaging have greatly facilitated the diagnosis and treatment of orbital tumors and pseudotumors. It is important for physicians to correctly diagnose orbital lesions so that appropriate therapeutic measures can be taken. We have designed this atlas to assist the clinician in that regard.

We have attempted to illustrate and discuss the clinical variations, histopathologic characteristics, and management of most orbital tumors and pseudotumors. Each specific entity is described in a concise review with pertinent references on the left-hand page and six color figures on the facing right-hand page, allowing the reader to obtain a complete uninterrupted overview of the subject without having to turn pages to find corresponding figures and references. This atlas is generously illustrated with 779 photographs and 25 drawings that depict the clinical and pathological variations and management of almost all lesions that are known to affect the orbit. It includes common lesions as well as some rare and fascinating conditions. It is rich in clinical, imaging, and pathologic correlations and clinical "pearls" based on our daily experience in the management of affected patients. Surgical principles are illustrated with high-quality professional colored drawings and photographs of the surgical procedures.

We hope that this unique atlas will benefit residents and fellows in ophthalmology, general ophthalmologists, ophthalmic subspecialists, and other practitioners who may evaluate patients with orbital tumors.

Jerry A. Shields, M.D.
Carol L. Shields, M.D.

Acknowledgments

A number of individuals have contributed directly or indirectly to the evolution and publication of this textbook. We are indebted to the many physicians in the United States and abroad who have referred to us their patients with orbital tumors. Their support of our subspecialty service has enabled us to improve our methods of diagnosis and treatment of patients with orbital tumors and to acquire the extensive collection of photographs that is used in this atlas.

We are particularly appreciative of our wonderful staff on the Oncology Service at Wills Eye Hospital of Thomas Jefferson University. Most of the slides used for photographs were organized and labeled in our department by Mary Ann Venditto, Sandra Dailey, Queen Warwick, Leslie Botti, and Marianne Pecora. We are especially grateful to our office manager, Bridget Walsh, for her continued support and enthusiasm. We also thank Kathy Smallenburg, Joann Delisi, Brenda Hall, Jacqueline Jurinich, Jeanine Ligon, Amia Scott, Christine Serlenga, and Tamicia Warrick for their assistance with patient care. We appreciate the continued support of the physicians and administrators at Wills Eye Hospital and Thomas Jefferson University.

Many of the excellent clinical photographs used in this atlas were taken by Terrance Tomer, Richard Lambert, Joyce Fellman, Robert Curtin, Jack Scully, and Roger Barone. We are deeply grateful to Robert Curtin and Jack Scully for taking numerous photographs in the operating room and for preparing and copying most of the slides used in the atlas.

We are truly indebted to our colleague and friend, Dr. Ralph C. Eagle, Jr. who over the years has spent many hours providing pathology consultations on our surgical cases. He also took many of the numerous gross photographs and photomicrographs of our patients that appear in this atlas. His talent for documenting photographically the fine details of ocular tumors is unparalleled. The numerous clinicopathologic correlations used in this atlas provide the reader with a better understanding of the ocular tumors.

Most of the photographs in this atlas are of patients whom we evaluated and managed personally, and it was not practical to acknowledge the referring physician in all cases. Some of the clinical and histopathologic photographs are from patients who were not evaluated personally by us but were taken from cases contributed by colleagues to the various ocular pathology societies and from articles published in the literature. In those instances, we have always attempted to give credit to the contributing physician.

We are grateful for the support of Christine Rullo, Paula Callaghan, Delois Patterson, Jonathan Geffner, David Dritsas, and their associates at Lippincott Williams & Wilkins for undertaking the publication of this atlas. With the generous help of these individuals and many others, the completion of this comprehensive atlas has been possible.

CHAPTER 1

Inflammatory Lesions That Simulate Neoplasms

DYSTHYROID ORBITOPATHY

There are a number of orbital inflammatory processes that are important in the differential diagnosis of orbital tumors. The most important of these are dysthyroid orbitopathy and idiopathic orbital inflammation ("inflammatory pseudotumor"). In addition, a number of bacterial, fungal, and idiopathic granulomatous diseases can cause orbital signs and symptoms.

Dysthyroid orbitopathy (Graves' disease, Graves' orbitopathy) is a common inflammatory condition that affects the extraocular muscles and has rather characteristic features. In some cases, it can simulate a neoplasm clinically and radiographically. The clinical features, diagnosis approaches, pathogenesis, pathology, and management are discussed in more detail in the literature (1–3) and only highlights are mentioned here.

Clinically, the patient with dysthyroid orbitopathy usually shows characteristic unilateral or bilateral proptosis, eyelid retraction, eyelid lag on down gaze, and conjunctival redness or edema. Computed tomography and magnetic resonance imaging show characteristic enlargement of rectus muscles with sparing of the muscle tendons and sparing of the orbital fat. Histopathology reveals infiltration of the affected muscles by lymphocytes. Severe complications include compressive optic neuropathy and exposure keratopathy. Depending on the severity of the disease and the complications, management can include observation, corticosteroids, radiotherapy, tarsorrhaphy, and orbital decompression.

SELECTED REFERENCES

1. Jakobiec FA, Jones IS. Orbital inflammations. In: Jones IS, Jakobiec FA, eds. *Diseases of the orbit.* Hagerstown, MD: Harper and Row, 1979:206–212.
2. Rootman J, Nugent R. Graves' orbitopathy. In: Rootman J, ed. *Diseases of the orbit.* Philadelphia: JB Lippincott Co., 1988:241–280.
3. Shields JA. *Diagnosis and management of orbital tumors.* Philadelphia: WB Saunders, 1989:69–72.

Dysthyroid Orbitopathy

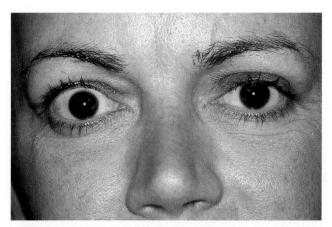

Figure 1-1. Dysthryoid orbitopathy with characteristic proptosis and eyelid retraction affecting mainly the right eye in a 35-year-old woman.

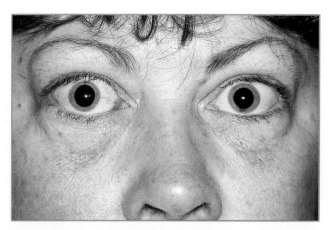

Figure 1-2. Dysthyroid orbitopathy with bilateral symmetric proptosis and eyelid retraction in a 43-year-old woman.

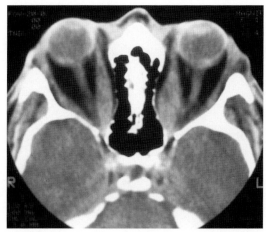

Figure 1-3. Axial computed tomography showing typical enlargement of extraocular muscles with sparing of the tendons. In this case, the medial rectus muscles mainly are involved.

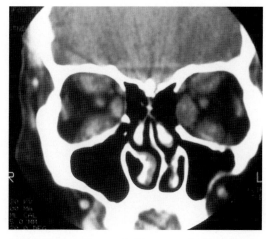

Figure 1-4. Coronal computed tomography through the midportion of the orbit showing enlargment of several rectus muscles.

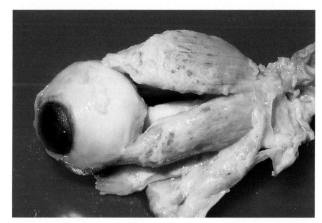

Figure 1-5. Gross specimen of globe and extraocular muscles removed postmortem from a patient with severe dysthyroid orbitopathy. Note the marked enlargement of all rectus muscles. (Courtesy of Dr. Ralph C. Eagle Jr.)

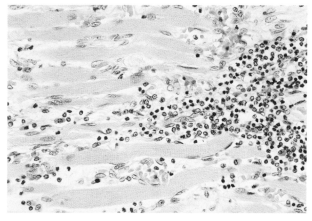

Figure 1-6. Histopathology of dysthyroid orbitopathy showing chronic inflammatory cells infiltrating the extraocular muscle (hematoxylin–eosin, original magnification × 100). (Courtesy of Dr. Ralph C. Eagle Jr.)

ACUTE ORBITAL CELLULITIS

Orbital cellulitis is an infection of the soft tissues posterior to the orbital septum (1,2). It is one of the most common causes of proptosis in children less than 5 years of age, in whom it most often is a complication of ethmoid sinusitis secondary to *Hemophilus influenza*. In older individuals, it is less common and can be due to a variety of organisms. In some instances, an orbital abscess can be localized and simulate a cyst or neoplasm. The patient generally presents with an abrupt onset of pain, eyelid edema, conjunctival hyperemia, and discharge. Treatment generally involves microscopic study and cultures of the discharge and appropriate antibiotic therapy. Surgical drainage is often helpful.

SELECTED REFERENCES

1. Rootman J, Robertson W, Lapointe JS. Orbital cellulitis. In: Rootman J, ed. *Diseases of the orbit.* Philadelphia: JB Lippincott Co., 1988:143–155.
2. Hornblass A, Herschorn BJ, Stern K, Grimes C. Orbital abscess. *Surv Ophthalmol* 1984;29:169–185.

Acute Orbital Cellulitis and Orbital Abscess

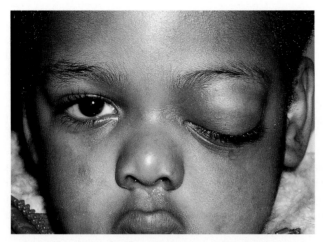

Figure 1-7. Acute orbital cellulitis secondary to ethmoid sinusitis and subperiosteal abscess in a 3-year-old child showing eyelid swelling and blepharoptosis.

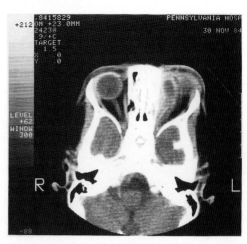

Figure 1-8. Axial computed tomography of the patient shown in Fig. 1-7 demonstrating ethmoiditis and left subperiosteal abscess.

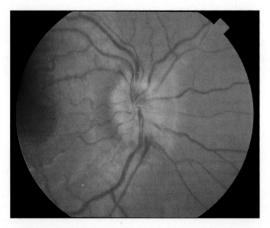

Figure 1-9. Fundus photograph showing edema and hyperemia of the right optic disc in an 8-year-old girl with circumscribed orbital abscess compressing the optic nerve.

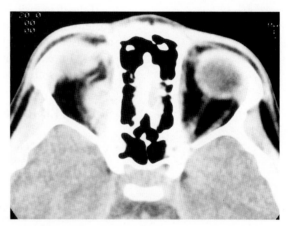

Figure 1-10. Axial computed tomography of the patient shown in Fig. 1-9 revealing circumscribed lesion in the orbit. The peripheral aspects of the lesion demonstrated gadolinium enhancement with magnetic resonance imaging.

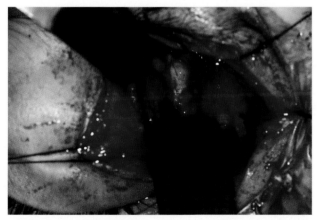

Figure 1-11. Surgical view of the lesion shown in Fig. 1-10, showing yellow purulent material coming from an abscess discovered at the time of surgical exploration. No organisms were found on stains and cultures.

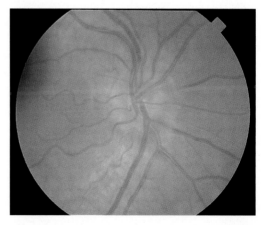

Figure 1-12. Appearance of the optic disc 2 months later. The disc edema resolved rapidly after drainage of the abscess and treatment with broad-spectrum antibiotics.

IDIOPATHIC ORBITAL INFLAMMATION ("INFLAMMATORY PSEUDOTUMOR")

Idiopathic orbital inflammation is a term used to describe a nongranulomatous inflammatory process within the orbit that has no recognizable local or systemic cause (1,2). There is considerable confusion regarding this condition, and the definition and classification most certainly will change as it is better understood and as more specific etiologies are identified.

The affected patient characteristically presents with an abrupt onset of ocular pain, proptosis, conjunctival chemosis, and sometimes visual impairment and diplopia. It can affect the orbit diffusely or it can affect specific tissues such as the lacrimal gland, extraocular muscles, or sclera. Involvement of each location can have specific manifestations on clinical examination and imaging studies. It usually affects adults but can occur in children, and it can be unilateral or bilateral (4). Findings on computed tomography and magnetic resonance imaging vary with the location and extent of involvement. The inflammatory process can extend throughout all soft tissues of the orbit, or it can produce an enhancing mass in the lacrimal gland, extraocular muscles, or other areas. The myositic type can be confined to one muscle (5,6). Histopathologically, the affected tissues are infiltrated by chronic inflammatory cells, mainly lymphocytes and plasma cells, without granulomatous inflammation. In children, there are generally more eosinophils. More chronic cases show marked fibrosis and sclerosis.

If the diagnosis is suspected clinically, the first course of management is oral corticosteroids in high doses followed by gradual tapering. Most cases show a dramatic response unless the lesion has extensive fibrosis. Steroid-resistant cases can be treated with cytotoxic agents or radiotherapy. Recurrence is common and a second course of treatment is often necessary (1,2).

SELECTED REFERENCES

1. Shields JA. *Diagnosis and management of orbital tumors.* Philadelphia: WB Saunders, 1989:72–75.
2. Rootman J, Robertson W, Lapointe JS. Inflammatory diseases. In: Rootman J, ed. *Diseases of the orbit.* Philadelphia: JB Lippincott Co., 1988:143–154.
3. Rootman J, Nugent R. The classification and management of acute orbital pseudotumors. *Ophthalmology* 1982;89:1040–1048.
4. Mottow LS, Jakobiec FA. Idiopathic inflammatory orbital pseudotumor in childhood. I. Clinical characteristics. *Arch Ophthalmol* 1978;96:1410–1416.
5. Mombaerts I, Koorneef L. Current status in the treatment of orbital myositis. *Ophthalmology* 1997;104:402–408.
6. Mannor GE, Rose GE, Moseley IF, Wright JE. Outcome of orbital myositis. Clinical features associated with recurrence. *Ophthalmology* 1997;104:409–414.

Idiopathic Orbital Inflammation in Adulthood

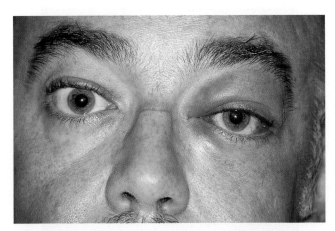

Figure 1-13. Acute orbital inflammation. Proptosis, eyelid edema, and conjunctival hyperemia in a 48-year-old man with acute ocular pain and visual loss.

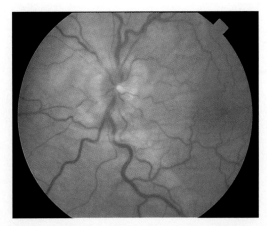

Figure 1-14. Fundus appearance of the left eye of the patient shown in Fig. 1-15 demonstrating edema of the optic disc secondary to compression of the optic nerve.

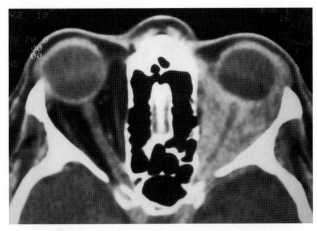

Figure 1-15. Axial computed tomography of the patient shown in Fig. 1-15 demonstrating diffuse involvement of all orbital tissues with compression of the optic nerve.

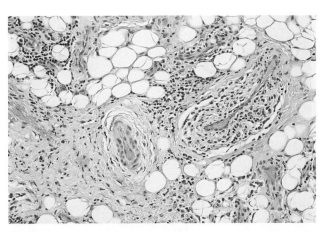

Figure 1-16. Histopathology of the mass shown in Fig. 1-15 demonstrating chronic nongranulomatous inflammation in the orbital fat (hematoxylin–eosin, original magnification × 50).

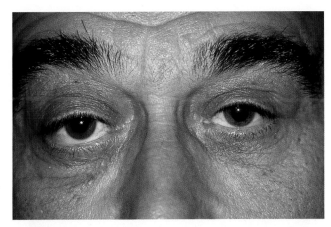

Figure 1-17. Chronic orbital inflammation. Bilateral proptosis in a 57-year-old man with chronic low-grade ocular pain.

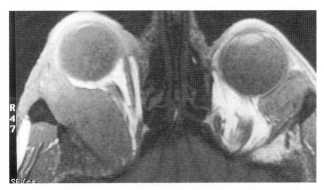

Figure 1-18. Axial magnetic resonance imaging of the patient shown in Fig. 1-13. Note the masses involving the lacrimal glands, lateral rectus muscles, and adjacent soft tissues. Histopathologic examination of the biopsy specimen confirmed the diagnosis of sclerosing idiopathic inflammation.

Idiopathic Orbital Inflammation in Childhood

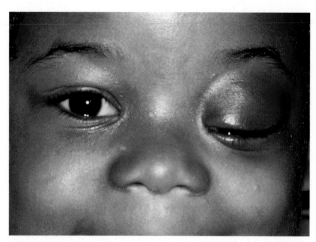

Figure 1-19. Acute swelling and ptosis of the left upper eyelid in a 4-year-old child.

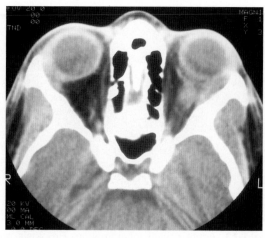

Figure 1-20. Axial computed tomography showing diffuse inflammation of the left orbit.

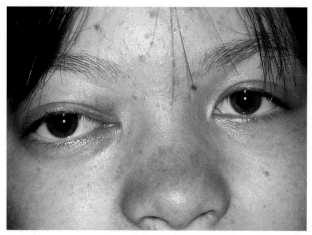

Figure 1-21. Proptosis and lateral displacement of the right eye in a 12-year-old girl with eyelid edema and mild pain.

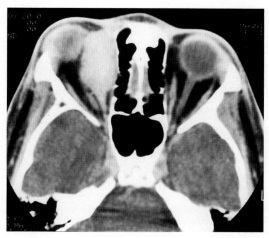

Figure 1-22. Axial computed tomography showing involvement of medial orbital tissues, mainly the medial rectus muscle.

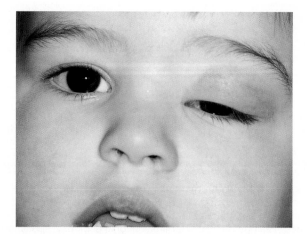

Figure 1-23. Proptosis, eyelid edema, and eyelid hyperemia in a 2-year-old child.

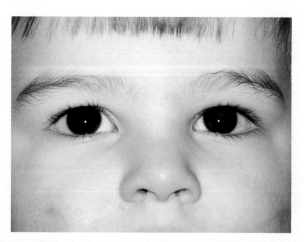

Figure 1-24. Appearance of the same child shortly after initiating a course of oral corticosteroids showing dramatic response.

Idiopathic Acute Orbital Myositis

This is a variant of acute nonspecific orbital inflammation that exclusively affects the extraocular muscles, often one specific muscle. The preferred treatment is systemic corticosteroids, and recurrences are common. Radiotherapy may not be effective in preventing recurrence.

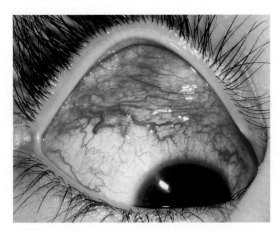

Figure 1-25. Acute redness secondary to a mass in superior epibulbar tissues in an 8-year-old boy. Rhabdomyosarcoma was a diagnostic consideration and a biopsy was done.

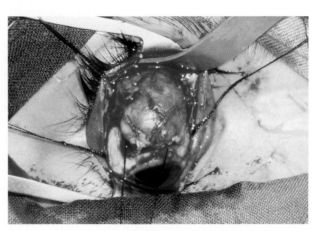

Figure 1-26. Surgical view of the area shown in Fig. 1-25. Note that a suture has been placed beneath the superior rectus and the exposed mass appears to involve the muscle itself. Histopathology revealed nongranulomatous inflammation.

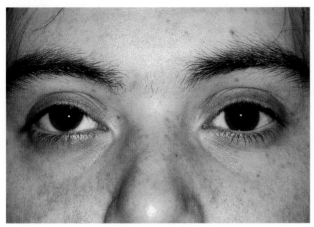

Figure 1-27. Proptosis of the right eye and blepharoptosis of the right upper eyelid in a 17-year-old boy.

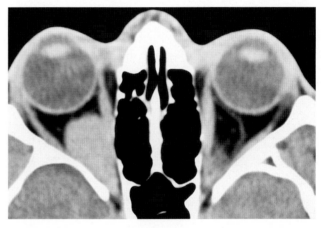

Figure 1-28. Axial computed tomography of the patient shown in Fig. 1-27. Note the smooth mass that appears to be in the muscle cone. Coronal computed tomographic studies showed the mass to correspond to an enlarged inferior rectus muscle.

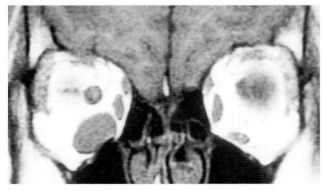

Figure 1-29. Coronal magnetic resonance imaging showing enlarged right inferior rectus muscle. Systemic corticosteroids were given.

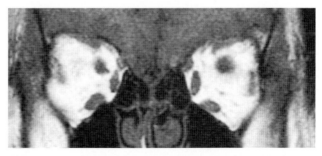

Figure 1-30. Coronal magnetic resonance imaging done 3 weeks later. There was a dramatic clinical response.

TUBERCULOSIS AND MUCORMYCOSIS

There are a number of inflammatory conditions that can affect the orbit (1–4). In some instances, a specific etiology, such as orbital foreign body or a mycotic or bacterial organism, can be identified. In many granulomatous inflammatory processes, such as sarcoidosis, Wegener's granulomatosis, Kimura's disease, and certain xanthogranulomas, a specific diagnosis can be applied based on the histopathologic pattern, but no specific etiology is recognized. Some granulomatous inflammations, such as xanthogranuloma, that affect mainly superficial structures, rather than the deeper orbital tissues, are discussed in more detail in the *Atlas of Eyelid and Conjunctival Tumors*.

Tuberculosis can occur as an isolated orbital or lacrimal gland granuloma, or it can extend into the orbit from the adjacent sinuses. It can be isolated to the orbital area, or it can be associated with pulmonary or extrapulmonary tuberculosis. Histopathologically, it occurs as a caseating granuloma with characteristic Langhan's giant cells. The diagnosis can be made by appropriate systemic evaluation and orbital biopsy. Treatment includes appropriate antituberculous therapy (3).

Mucormycosis (phycomycosis) is perhaps the best known of the orbital mycoses. It generally occurs in patients who have advanced disease, such as diabetic ketoacidosis, malignancies, or other conditions associated with immunosuppression. The diagnosis is made by clinical suspicion in the clinical settings and an orbital biopsy. The management is somewhat controversial and ranges from wide surgical debridement, which sometimes includes sino-orbital exenteration, and appropriate antifungal agents such as amphotericin B.

SELECTED REFERENCES

1. Shields JA. *Diagnosis and management of orbital tumors.* Philadelphia: WB Saunders, 1989:80–83.
2. Rootman J, Robertson W, Lapointe JS. Inflammatory diseases. In: Rootman J, ed. *Diseases of the orbit.* Philadelphia: JB Lippincott Co., 1988:143–154.
3. Khalil MK, Lindley S, Matouk E. Tuberculosis of the orbit. *Ophthalmology* 1985;92:1624–1627.
4. Obenauf CD, Shaw HE, Sydnor CF, et al. Sarcoidosis and its ophthalmic manifestations. *Am J Ophthalmol* 1978;86:648–655.

Orbital Tuberculosis and Mucormycosis

Figs.1-33 and 1-34 courtesy of Dr. Mourad Khalil. From Khalil MK, Lindley S, Matouk E. Tuberculosis of the orbit. *Ophthalmology* 1985;92:1624–1627.

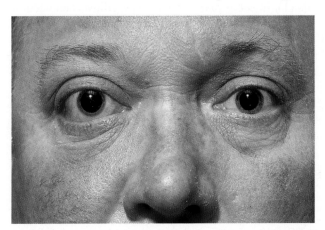

Figure 1-31. Proptosis of the right eye in an otherwise healthy 51-year-old man.

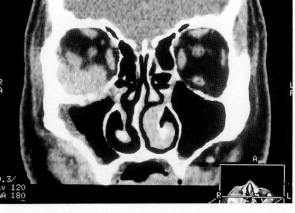

Figure 1-32. Coronal computed tomography of the patient shown in Fig. 1-31 depicting diffuse mass in the inferior and posterior aspects of the orbit. Biopsy showed granulomatous inflammation and acid-fast organisms compatible with tuberculosis or atypical mycobacteria.

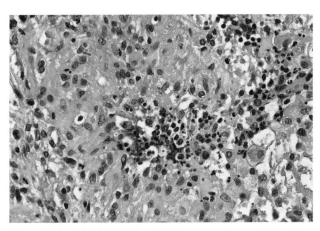

Figure 1-33. Histopathology of the lesion shown in Fig. 1-32, revealing histiocytes within a necrotizing granuloma (hematoxylin–eosin, original magnification × 150).

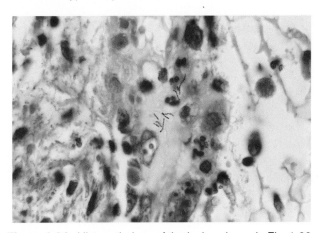

Figure 1-34. Histopathology of the lesion shown in Fig. 1-32, demonstrating acid-fast organisms in a giant cell (acid-fast stain, original magnification × 1,000).

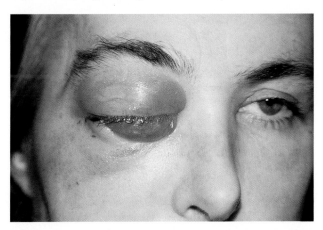

Figure 1-35. Proptosis and redness and swelling of eyelids on the right side secondary to orbital mucormycosis in a 41-year-old woman with diabetes mellitus and chronic debilitation secondary to presumed Weber–Christian disease. Biopsy revealed mucormycosis. (Courtesy of Dr. James Powell.)

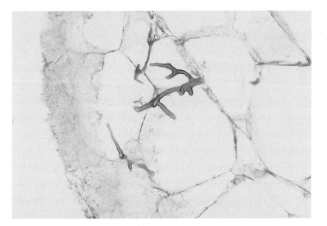

Figure 1-36. Histopathology of orbital mucormycosis showing characteristic organisms (periodic acid–Schiff × 200). (Courtesy of Dr. George Howard.)

ORBITAL ASPERGILLOSIS—ALLERGIC FUNGAL SINUSITIS

Aspergillosis is another important mycotic infection that can involve the orbit. Unlike mucormycosis, which occurs in debilitated patients, aspergillosis often occurs in otherwise healthy individuals (1). In some cases, orbital aspergillosis can occur as allergic fungal sinusitis (AFS). AFS is a disease characterized by recurrent sinusitis, eosinophilia, and increased serum immunoglobulin E levels. Patients are typically young and have a history of asthma and nasal polyposis. Orbital involvement by AFS has been recognized with increasing frequency in recent years. Computed tomography shows a mass in the sinuses with secondary unilateral or bilateral orbital extension. Histopathology shows sloughing of necrotic epithelial cells with extensive mucous and degenerating eosinophils, often with Charcot–Leyden crystals. In neglected cases, orbital aspergillosis can be fatal (1–4).

SELECTED REFERENCES

1. Shields JA. *Diagnosis and management of orbital tumors.* Philadelphia: WB Saunders, 1989:80–83.
2. Chang W, Shields CL, Shields JA, Eagle RC, Nelson LB, DePotter P. Bilateral orbital involvement with massive allergic fungal sinusitis. *Arch Ophthalmol* 1966;114:767–768.
3. Hutnik CML, Nicolle DA, Munoz DG. Orbital aspergillosis. A fatal masquerader. *J Neuro-Ophthalmol* 1997;17:257–261.
4. Klapper SR, Lee AG, Patrinely JR, Stewart M, Alford ELK. Orbital involvement in allergic fungal sinusitis. *Ophthalmology* 1997;104:2094–2100.

Orbital Involvement with Allergic Fungal Sinusitis due to Aspergillosis

Depicted is a clinicopathologic correlation of allergic fungal sinusitis in an 11-year-old girl.

From Chang W, Shields CL, Shields JA, Eagle RC, Nelson LB, DePotter P. Bilateral orbital involvement with massive allergic fungal sinusitis. *Arch Ophthalmol* 1996;114: 767–768.

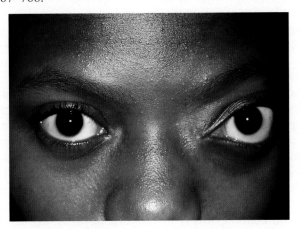

Figure 1-37. Proptosis of the left eye in an 11-year-old girl.

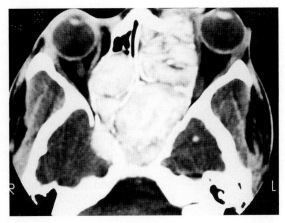

Figure 1-38. Axial computed tomography showing contrast-enhancing soft-tissue lesion filling and expanding the ethmoid sinus, sphenoid sinus, and nasal cavity and encroaching on both orbits.

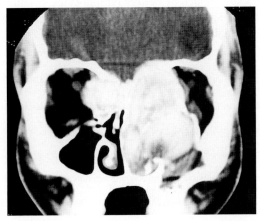

Figure 1-39. Axial computed tomography further demonstrating the extent of the lesion.

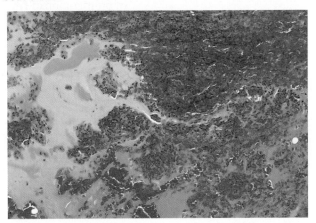

Figure 1-40. Biopsy specimen showing amorphous necrotic tissue and chronic inflammatory cells (hematoxylin–eosin, original magnification × 50). Cultures taken at surgery demonstrated *Aspergillus flavus*.

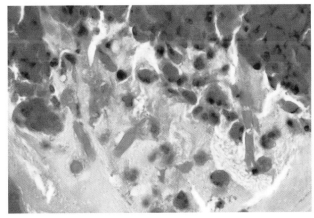

Figure 1-41. Higher magnification photomicrograph showing fungi (hematoxylin–eosin, original magnification × 200).

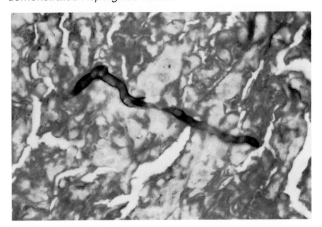

Figure 1-42. Fungus stain demonstrating the organisms. (Gomori methenamine silver × 250).

IDIOPATHIC GRANULOMATOUS INFLAMMATION OF THE ORBIT

Considered here are some selected idiopathic granulomatous inflammations including sarcoidosis, Wegener's granulomatosis, and Kimura's disease.

Sarcoidosis is a systemic disease of unknown etiology characterized by subacute or chronic inflammation involving lungs, liver, spleen, skin bone marrow, and ocular structures. It is more common in black patients. In the orbit, it generally occurs as a solitary granuloma that frequently is confined to the lacrimal gland, unilaterally or bilaterally. Elevated serum angiotensin-converting enzyme is strongly suggestive of the clinical diagnosis. Histopathologically, there is noncaseating granulomatous inflammation with giant cells. Biopsy usually is done to confirm the diagnosis and treatment is systemic corticosteroids (1–3).

Wegener's granulomatosis is a multisystem disease consisting of necrotizing granulomas and vasculitis of the respiratory tract, generalized small-vessel vasculitis, and focal necrotizing glomerulonephritis. It can involve the orbit as a part of widespread disease or as limited form without the characteristic renal involvement (4). Positive titers for antineutrophil cytoplasmic antibody is helpful in establishing the diagnosis. Histopathology shows granulomatous inflammation with multinucleated giant cells and necrotizing vasculitis. Management is systemic corticosteroids or cyclophosphamide.

Angiolymphoid hyperplasia with eosinophilia (Kimura's disease) is an idiopathic inflammation of the skin that typically involves the head and neck area (5). Orbital involvement can occur as a localized or diffuse process. Most cases are unilateral, but bilateral involvement often occurs (6). Histopathologically, it consists of a central area of proliferation of fine blood vessels surrounded by benign lymphocytes, plasma cells, and eosinophils. Most cases are managed by surgical excision, but systemic corticosteroids should be considered for residual orbital tissue.

SELECTED REFERENCES

1. Shields JA. *Diagnosis and management of orbital tumors.* Philadelphia: WB Saunders, 1989:75–78.
2. Obenauf CD, Shaw HE, Sydnor CF, Klintworth GK. Sarcoidosis and its ophthalmic manifestations. *Am J Ophthalmol* 1978;86:648–655.
3. Cornblath WT, Elner V, Rolfe M. Extraocular muscle involvement in sarcoidosis. *Ophthalmology* 1993;100: 501–505.
4. Bullen CL, Liesegang TJ, McDonald TJ, DeRemme RA. Ocular complications of Wegener's granulomatosis. *Ophthalmology* 1983;90:279–290.
5. Hidayat AA, Cameron DJ, Fong RL, et al. Angiolymphoid hyperplasia with eosinophilia (Kimura's disease) of the orbit and ocular adnexa. *Am J Ophthalmol* 1983;96:176–189.
6. Shields CL, Shields JA, Glass RM. Bilateral orbital involvement in angiolymphoid hyperplasia with eosinophilia. Kimura's disease. *Orbit* 1990;9:89–95.

Orbital Sarcoidosis

Orbital sarcoidosis most often involves the lacrimal gland. Less commonly it affects extraocular muscles or other orbital tissues. Depicted is a case involving the lacrimal gland and a case involving extraocular muscle.

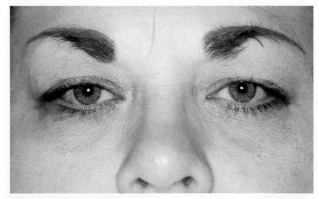

Figure 1-43. Swelling of temporal aspect of the right upper eyelid in a 42-year-old woman. Systemic evaluation was unrevealing and angiotensin-converting enzyme level was normal. (Courtesy of Drs. Daniel Albert, Morton Smith, and Nasreen Syed.)

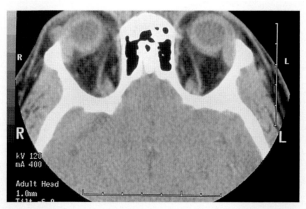

Figure 1-44. Axial computed tomography of the patient shown in Fig. 1-43 demonstrating an irregular mass in the right lacrimal gland. (Courtesy of Drs. Daniel Albert, Morton Smith, and Nasreen Syed.)

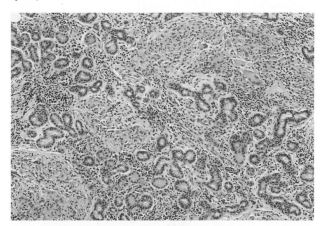

Figure 1-45. Histopathology of the lesion shown in Fig. 1-44 showing noncaseating granuloma compatible with sarcoidosis involving the lacrimal gland (hematoxylin–eosin, original magnification × 50). (Courtesy of Drs. Daniel Albert, Morton Smith, and Nasreen Syed.)

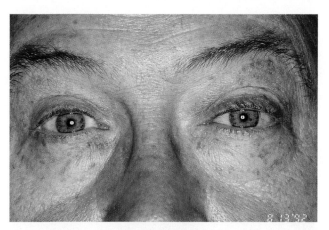

Figure 1-46. Swelling of the right upper eyelid and slight left proptosis in a 47-year-old man with a history of pulmonary sarcoidosis and a highly positive angiotensin-converting enzyme value. (Courtesy of Drs. Ronan Conlon and Keith Carter.)

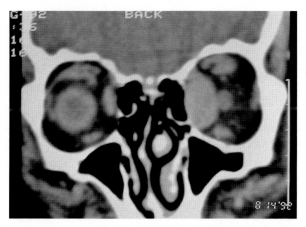

Figure 1-47. Coronal computed tomography of the patient shown in Fig. 1-46 revealing circumscribed enlargement of the medial rectus muscle. (Courtesy of Drs. Ronan Conlon and Keith Carter.)

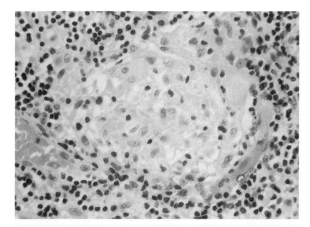

Figure 1-48. Photomicrograph of the lesion shown in Fig. 1-46 demonstrating a noncaseating epitheliod cell granuloma (hematoxylin–eosin, original magnification × 250). (Courtesy of Drs. Ronan Conlon and Keith Carter.)

Orbital Involvement with Wegener's Granulomatosis

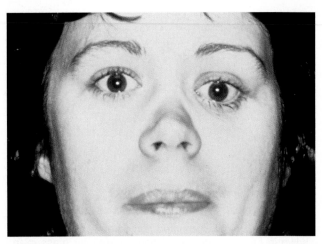

Figure 1-49. Slight proptosis of the right eye in a 28-year-old woman with diplopia and slight visual impairment in the right eye. (Courtesy of Dr. Curtis Margo.)

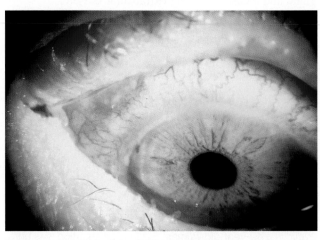

Figure 1-50. Epibulbar findings of diffuse scleritis and a peripheral gutter-like corneal ulcer in the patient shown in Fig. 1-49, characteristic features of Wegener's granulomatosis. (Courtesy of Dr. Curtis Margo.)

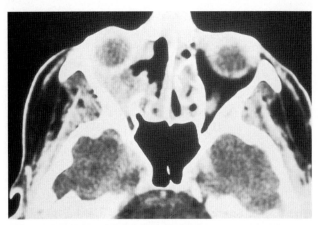

Figure 1-51. Axial computed tomography of same patient near inferior aspect of globes, showing diffuse mass and bone destruction nasally near the orbital apex. (Courtesy of Dr. Curtis Margo.)

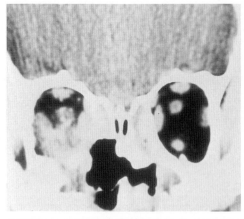

Figure 1-52. Coronal computed tomography showing diffuse mass and bone destruction in floor of orbit. Orbital biopsy showed findings consistent with Wegener's granulomatosis. (Courtesy of Dr. Curtis Margo.)

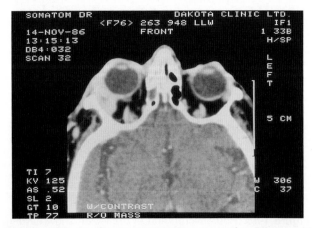

Figure 1-53. Axial computed tomography of a 70-year-old woman with a limited form of Wegener's granulomatosis. Note the mass in the vicinity of the lateral rectus muscle. (Courtesy of Dr. Jerry Kobrin.)

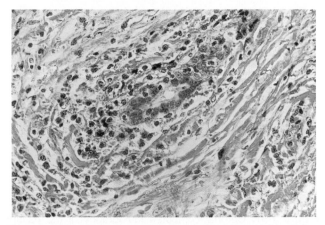

Figure 1-54. Histopathology of the lesion depicted in Fig. 1-53 showing necrotizing vasculitis (hematoxylin–eosin, original magnification × 100). (Courtesy of Dr. Jerry Kobrin.)

Orbital Involvement with Kimura's Disease

A clinicopathologic correlation of orbital involvement with angiolymphoid hyperplasia with eosinophilia (Kimura's disease) is depicted. This case is atypical because of the bilateral involvement. Most cases are unilateral.

From Shields CL, Shields JA, Glass RM. Bilateral orbital involvement in angiolymphoid hyperplasia with eosinophilia. Kimura's disease. *Orbit* 1990;9:89–95.

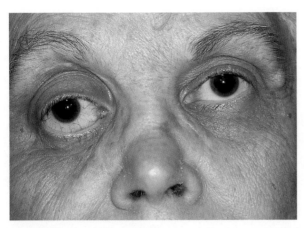

Figure 1-55. Proptosis and downward displacement of the right eye in a 55-year-old woman.

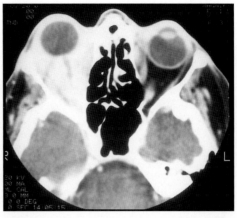

Figure 1-56. Axial computed tomography showing massive involvement of soft tissue of the right orbit and less severe involvement of the left orbit.

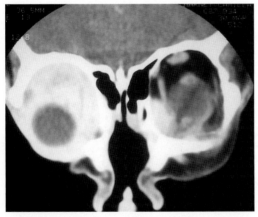

Figure 1-57. Coronal computed tomography showing marked involvement of the right orbit with less extensive involvement of the left orbit.

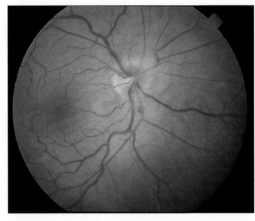

Figure 1-58. Fundus photograph of the right eye showing choroidal folds in the macular area secondary to the orbital mass.

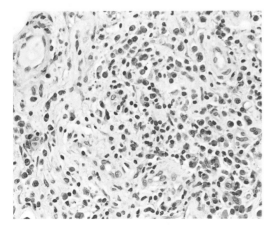

Figure 1-59. Photomicrograph of biopsy of the patient's right orbit showing granulomatous inflammation with blood vessels and numerous eosinophils (hematoxylin–eosin, original magnification × 75).

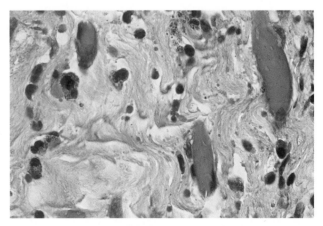

Figure 1-60. Photomicrograph of the same specimen shown in Fig. 1-59 demonstrating blood vessels, sclerosis, and eosinophils (hematoxylin–eosin, original magnification × 300).

CHAPTER 2

Cystic Lesions

DERMOID CYST

Dermoid cyst is the most common cystic lesion in the orbit. It is a congenital lesion that forms from epithelial cells that are entrapped during embryogenesis beneath the surface epithelium, often near bony sutures (1–6). It most often occurs near the orbital rim superotemporally at the zygomaticofrontal suture, but it can occur at the site of other bony sutures and in the deeper orbital soft tissue. In some instances, a dermoid cyst can have extraorbital and intraorbital components that are connected through a defect in bone (dumbbell dermoid) (7). Imaging studies show a cystic lesion with enhancement of the wall but no significant enhancement of the lumen.

Histopathologically, the cyst is lined by surface epithelium (epidermis or conjunctiva). Cysts lined by conjunctival epithelium more often are found in the orbital soft tissue nasally (8,9). The cyst wall can contain dermal appendages, sebaceous glands, and sweat glands. The cyst lumen contains epithelial cells, sebaceous material, and hairs (2).

Management ranges from observation to surgical excision, with most being removed surgically because the patient presents with a cosmetically visible lesion or ocular symptoms due to rupture of the cyst and orbital inflammation. An anteriorly located orbital dermoid cyst can be excised via a cutaneous or conjunctival approach. A deeper cyst may require a lateral orbitotomy. Care should be taken to avoid surgical rupture of the cyst. If rupture occurs, vigorous irrigation and instillation of antibiotics or corticosteroids is advisable to prevent postoperative inflammation (6).

SELECTED REFERENCES

1. Shields JA. *Diagnosis and management of orbital tumors.* Philadelphia: WB Saunders, 1989:94–97.
2. Shields JA, Bakewell B, Augsburger DG, Flanagan CJ. Classification and incidence of space-occupying lesions of the orbit. A survey of 645 biopsies. *Arch Ophthalmol* 1984;102:1606–1611.
3. Sherman RP, Rootman J, Lapointe JJ. Orbital dermoids: clinical presentation and management. *Br J Ophthalmol* 1984;68:642–652.
4. Shields JA, Bakewell B, Augsburger DG, Donoso LA, Bernardino V. Space-occupying orbital masses in children. A review of 250 consecutive biopsies. *Ophthalmology* 1986;93:379–384.
5. Sathananthan N, Moseley IF, Rose GE, Wright JE. The frequency and clinical significance of bone involvement in outer canthus dermoid cysts. *Br J Ophthalmol* 1993;77:789–794.
6. Shields JA, Kaden IH, Eagle RC Jr, Shields CL. Orbital dermoid cysts. Clinicopathologic correlations, classification, and management. The 1997 Josephine E. Schueler Lecture. *Ophthal Plast Reconstr Surg* 1997;13:265–276.
7. Emerick GT, Shields CL, Shields JA, Eagle RC Jr, De Potter P, Markowitz GI. Chewing-induced visual impairment from a dumbbell dermoid cyst. *Ophthal Plast Reconstr Surg* 1997;13:57–61.
8. Jakobiec FA, Bonanno PA, Sigelman J. Conjunctival adnexal cysts and dermoids. *Arch Ophthalmol* 1978;96:1404–1409.
9. Shields JA, Augsburger JJ, Donoso LA. Orbital dermoid cyst of conjunctival origin. *Am J Ophthalmol* 1986;101:726–79.

Orbital Dermoid Cyst

Most dermoid cysts in the orbital region are located superotemporally near the zygomaticofrontal suture. A typical case with imaging, surgical approach, and pathology is shown.

From Shields JA, Kaden IH, Eagle RC Jr, Shields CL. Orbital dermoid cysts. Clinicopathologic correlations, classification, and management. The 1997 Josephine E. Schueler Lecture. *Ophthal Plast Reconstr Surg* 1997;13:265–276.

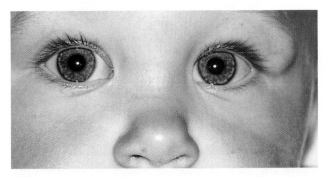

Figure 2-1. Characteristic subcutaneous mass superotemporal to the left eye in a 2-month-old boy.

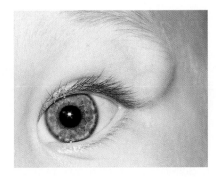

Figure 2-2. Closer view of the same lesion shown in Fig. 2-1.

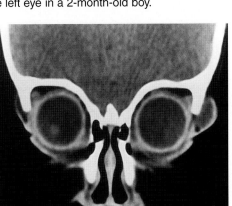

Figure 2-3. Coronal computed tomogram in T1-weighted image showing cystic lesion at the orbital rim. The lumen of the cyst shows features similar to vitreous and orbital fat.

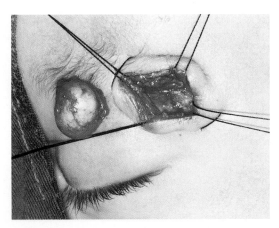

Figure 2-4. The cyst (to the *left*) has been removed by a cutaneous approach. One can use either an infrabrow or eyelid crease incision. The posterior aspect of the cyst is often adherent to the periosteum, requiring meticulous dissection to remove the cyst intact.

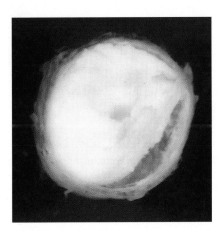

Figure 2-5. Gross appearance of the cyst after fixation and sectioning. Note the capsule and the yellow material in the lumen.

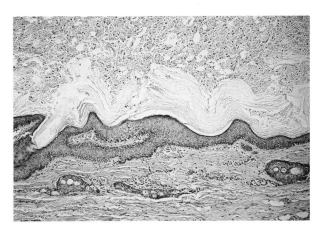

Figure 2-6. Histopathology through the cyst wall (*bottom*) and the lumen (*top*). The cyst is lined by keratinizing epithelium and has dermal elements in the wall and in the lumen.

Dermoid Cyst of Conjunctival Origin

Dermoid cysts that are lined by conjunctival epithelium usually occur in the orbital soft tissues nasally (1–3). They may derive from primitive epithelium destined to form the adult caruncle. A clinicopathologic correlation is shown.

From Shields JA, Augsburger JJ, Donoso LA. Orbital dermoid cyst of conjunctival origin. *Am J Ophthalmol* 1986;101:726–729.

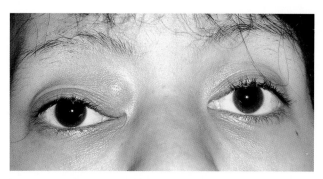

Figure 2-7. Soft-tissue subcutaneous mass superonasally on the right side in a 17-year-old girl.

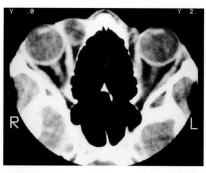

Figure 2-8. Axial computed tomogram showing the cystic nature of the lesion.

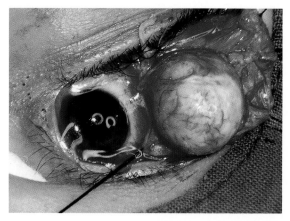

Figure 2-9. Cyst has been exposed and removed through a superonasal conjunctival approach.

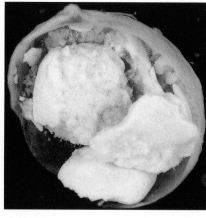

Figure 2-10. Gross appearance of the cyst after fixation and sectioning. Note the very thin capsule and the yellow material in the lumen.

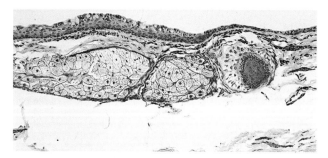

Figure 2-11. Photomicrograph showing wall of the cyst with nonkeratinizing epithelium, hair shafts, and sebaceous glands (hematoxylin–eosin, original magnification × 25).

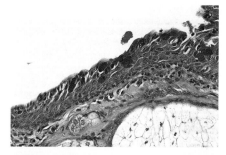

Figure 2-12. Photomicrograph showing wall of the cyst with nonkeratinizing epithelium containing periodic acid–Schiff-positive goblet cells (periodic acid–Schiff, original magnification × 50).

Dermoid Cyst of Conjunctival Origin in an Adult

Although orbital dermoid cysts are congenital, the soft-tissue dermoid cyst of conjunctival origin may lie dormant for many years before clinical detection. Such cysts have been recognized in patients more than 70 years old. A clinicopathologic correlation in a 50-year-old patient is shown.

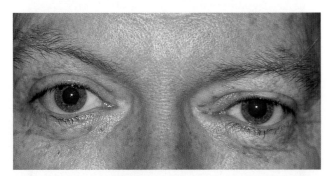

Figure 2-13. Slight blepharoptosis and inferotemporal displacement of the left eye.

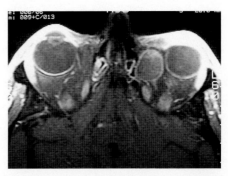

Figure 2-14. Axial magnetic resonance imaging showing temporal displacement of the left eye by a cystic mass.

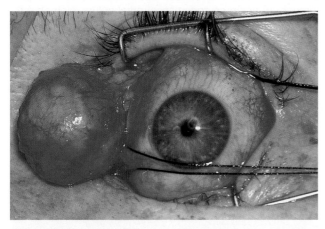

Figure 2-15. Lesion being removed intact via a forniceal incision in the conjunctiva.

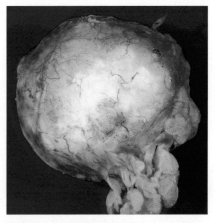

Figure 2-16. Gross appearance of the intact cyst after excision. Note the yellow material deep to the thin capsule.

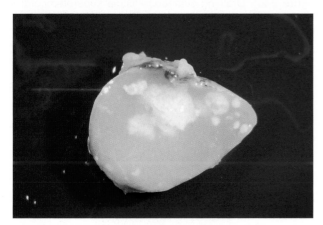

Figure 2-17. Gross appearance of the cyst after fixation and sectioning. Note the very thin capsule and the yellow material in the lumen.

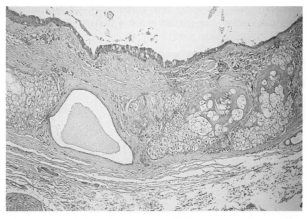

Figure 2-18. Histopathology through the cyst wall (*bottom*) and the lumen (*top*). The cyst is lined by keratinizing epithelium and has dermal elements in the wall and in the lumen (hematoxylin–eosin, original magnification × 40).

Orbital Dermoid Cysts—Dumbbell Type

Dumbbell cysts are characterized by two cystic components connected by a channel through the adjacent bone, at the site of a bony suture. Like other subcutaneous dermoid cysts, they can break through the epidermis and produce a draining fistula.

Figs. 2-19 through 2-21 from Emerick GT, Shields CL, Shields JA, Eagle RC Jr, De Potter P, Markowitz GI. Chewing-induced visual impairment from a dumbbell dermoid cyst. *Ophthal Plast Reconstr Surg* 1997;13:57–61.

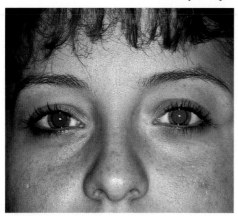

Figure 2-19. Subcutaneous mass temporal to the left eye in a 29-year-old woman.

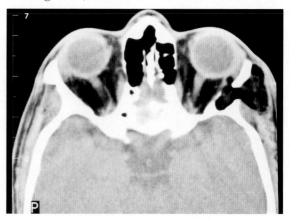

Figure 2-20. Axial computed tomogram of the patient shown in Fig. 2-19 showing bilobed cystic lesion communicating through an enlarged zygomaticofrontal suture. Note that the lumen of the lesion is similar to vitreous and orbital fat. The lesion was excised in piecemeal fashion.

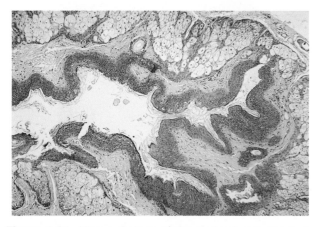

Figure 2-21. Histopathology of the excised cyst shown in Fig. 2-20 demonstrating the keratinizing epithelium with numerous sebaceous glands in the wall (hematoxylin–eosin, original magnification × 40).

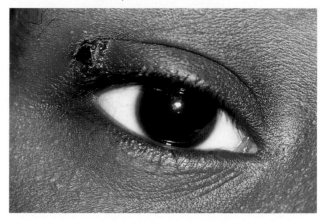

Figure 2-22. Draining cutaneous fistula superotemporal to the right eye in an 8-year-old boy. Such a fistula in this location is highly suggestive of a ruptured dermoid cyst.

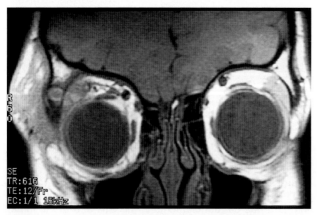

Figure 2-23. Coronal magnetic resonance imaging in T1-weighted image of the patient shown in Fig. 2-22 revealing the bony defect connecting the two lobes.

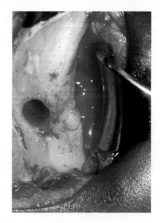

Figure 2-24. Osseous defect seen at time of surgery after piecemeal removal of the dermoid cyst.

Deep Orbital Dermoid Cyst

Large dermoid cysts located in the posterior orbit pose more of a diagnostic and therapeutic challenge. Such cysts can grow slowly to a large size at a young age and can recur after excision. A clinicopathologic correlation is depicted.

From Leonardo D, Shields CL, Shields JA, Nelson LB. Recurrent giant orbital dermoid of infancy. *J Pediatr Ophthalmol Strabismus* 1994;31:50–52.

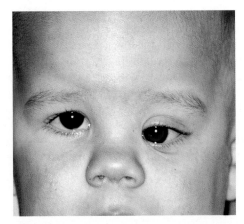

Figure 2-25. Proptosis and downward displacement of the the left eye in a 2-year-old boy. The findings were noted shortly after birth and had become progressively worse.

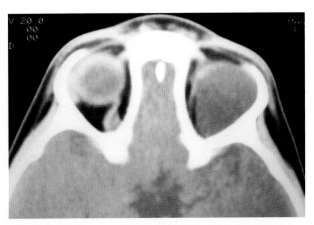

Figure 2-26. Axial computed tomogram showing large superior orbital mass.

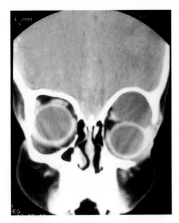

Figure 2-27. Coronal computed tomogram showing mass above the globe. Note that the orbit is larger and there is superior displacement of the orbital roof.

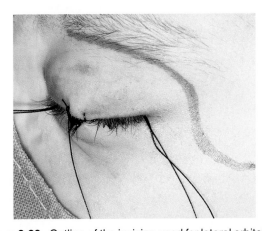

Figure 2-28. Outline of the incision used for lateral orbitotomy.

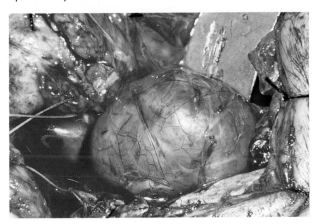

Figure 2-29. Cystic mass exposed after lateral orbitotomy. It was aspirated and removed.

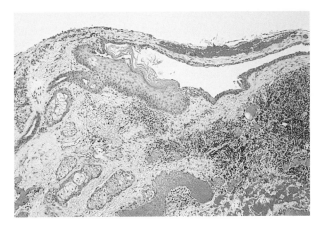

Figure 2-30. Histopathology of a portion of the collapsed cyst showing features of a dermoid cyst. Although most of the cyst was lined by nonkeratinizing epithelium similar to conjunctiva, a small portion of it showed keratinizing epithelium. The lesion recurred in the temporal orbit about 2 years later and was excised surgically with a good result.

CONJUNCTIVAL EPITHELIAL CYST

Epithelial cysts in the orbital area can be lined by cutaneous epithelium (epidermis), conjunctival epithelium, respiratory epithelium, or occasionally other epithelial structures. Primary cutaneous epithelial cyst (epidermoid cyst) is more common in the eyebrow and eyelid region and is discussed in the *Atlas of Eyelid and Conjunctival Tumors*. A conjunctival epithelial cyst is characterized by a lining of epithelial cells with features of conjunctiva but without dermal appendages, a feature that distinguishes it from a conjunctival dermoid cyst described in the prior section (1–4). A conjunctival epithelial cyst can occur spontaneously with no apparent etiology but, more often, it occurs following surgery such as strabismus surgery, retinal detachment surgery, and enucleation (5,6). It more commonly occurs in subconjunctival tissues, but it can occur in the anterior orbital tissues. In such instances, conjunctival epithelium that predisposes to the cyst probably is implanted into the orbital tissues at the time of the surgery. Simple conjunctival epithelial cyst occasionally is seen with chronic inflammation (7).

SELECTED REFERENCE

1. Shields JA. *Diagnosis and management of orbital tumors.* Philadelphia: WB Saunders, 1989:94–97.
2. Henderson JW. *Orbital tumors*, 3rd ed. New York: Raven Press, 1994:53–61.
3. Jakobiec FA, Bonanno PA, Sigelman J. Conjunctival adnexal cysts and dermoids. *Arch Ophthalmol* 1978;96: 1404–1409.
4. Boynton JR, Searl SS, Ferry AP, et al. Primary nonkeratinized epithelial ("conjunctival") orbital cysts. *Arch Ophthalmol* 1992;110:1238–1242.
5. Johnson DW, Bartley GB, Garrity JA, Robertson DM. Massive epithelium-lined cyst after scleral buckling. *Am J Ophthalmol* 1992;113:439–444.
6. De Potter P, Kunin AW, Shields CL, Shields JA, Nase PK. Massive orbital cyst of the lateral rectus muscle after retinal detachment surgery. *Ophthal Plast Reconstr Surg* 1993;9:292–297.
7. Desai V, Shields CL, Shields JA. Orbital cyst in a patient with Stevens–Johnson syndrome. *Cornea* 1992;11: 592–594.

Orbital Conjunctival Epithelial Cyst Following Enucleation

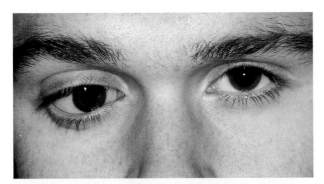

Figure 2-31. Downward displacement and proptosis of the enucleation prosthesis in an 18-year-old man who underwent enucleation for retinoblastoma 16 years earlier.

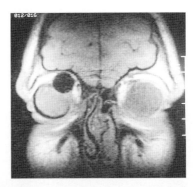

Figure 2-32. Coronal magnetic resonance imaging showing a large cyst, the size of a normal globe, displacing the silastic ball implant superonasally.

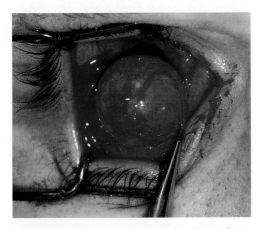

Figure 2-33. View of the implant at the time of surgery to remove the cyst.

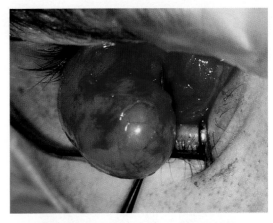

Figure 2-34. View of the large cyst that is being removed after the implant was taken out.

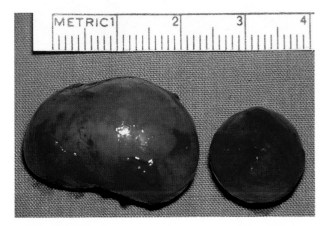

Figure 2-35. Appearance of cyst (to the *left*) and the removed implant (to the *right*) immediately after surgical removal.

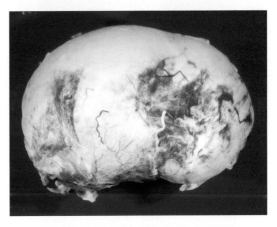

Figure 2-36. Gross view of the cyst after fixation.

Orbital Conjunctival Epithelial Cyst Following Retinal Detachment Surgery

An orbital cyst can develop after retinal detachment surgery, presumably from displacement of conjunctival epithelium into the deeper orbital tissues. A clinicopathologic correlation is shown.

From De Potter P, Kunin AW, Shields CL, Shields JA, Nase PK. Massive orbital cyst of the lateral rectus muscle after retinal detachment surgery. *Ophthal Plast Reconstr Surg* 1993;9:292–297.

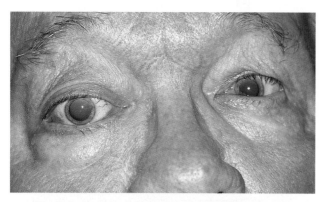

Figure 2-37. Proptosis of the right eye in a 76-year-old man who had undergone ipsilateral retinal detachment surgery several years earlier.

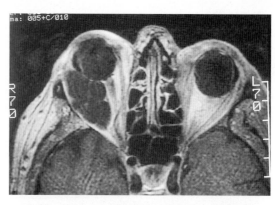

Figure 2-38. Axial magnetic resonance imaging in T1-weighted image showing an irregular cyst in the lateral portion of the orbit.

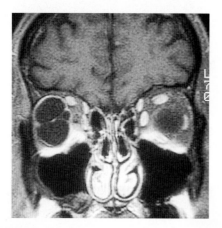

Figure 2-39. Coronal magnetic resonance imaging in T1-weighted image showing the cyst.

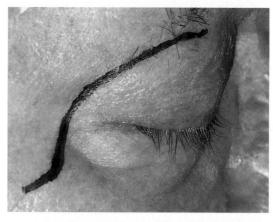

Figure 2-40. Outline of the superotemporal orbitotomy incision used to remove the cyst.

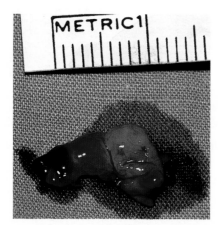

Figure 2-41. A portion of the collapsed cyst shown after it was aspirated and removed in a piecemeal fashion.

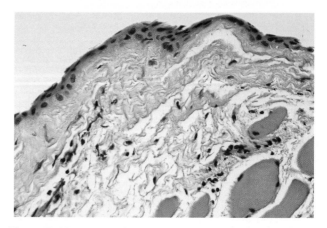

Figure 2-42. Histopathology of the wall of the cyst showing nonkeratinizing epithelium.

Orbital Conjunctival Epithelial Cyst Associated with Stevens–Johnson Syndrome

It is possible that adhesions between the tarsal and bulbar conjunctiva can entrap conjunctival epithelium and lead to a cyst. That may have been the mechanism in the case shown below.

From Desai V, Shields CL, Shields JA. Orbital cyst in a patient with Stevens–Johnson syndrome. *Cornea* 1992;11:592–594.

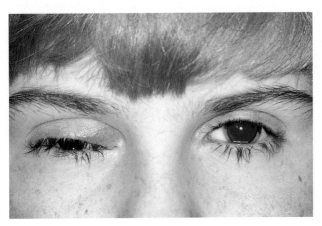

Figure 2-43. Blepharoptosis and an irritated, uncomfortable right eye in a 10-year-old girl who had Stevens–Johnson syndrome with severe ocular involvement. The cyst had recurred after simple aspiration.

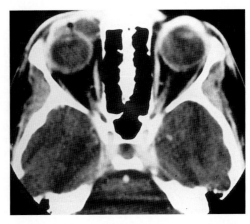

Figure 2-44. Axial computed tomogram showing cystic lesion superior and nasal to the globe.

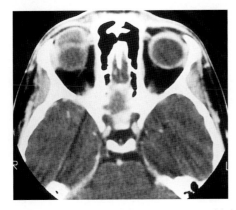

Figure 2-45. Axial computed tomogram at a higher level showing extent of the cyst.

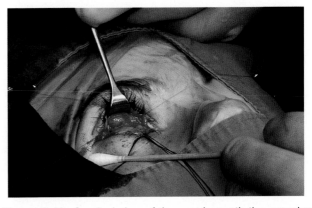

Figure 2-46. Surgical view of the cyst beneath the superior fornix. The cyst was removed and a buccal mucous membrane graft was done.

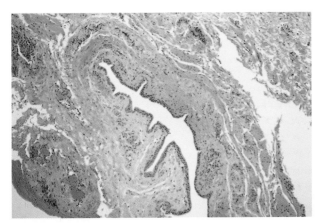

Figure 2-47. Histopathology showing fibrotic wall secondary to chronic inflammation (hematoxylin–eosin, original magnification × 10).

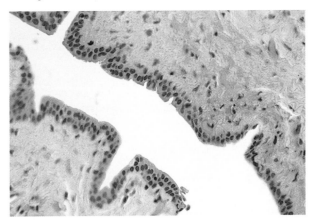

Figure 2-48. Histopathology showing nonkeratinizing epithelium (hematoxylin–eosin, original magnification × 30).

TERATOMA

Teratoma is a tumor that contains elements of the three embryonic germ layers. It occasionally involves the orbit, where it can cause pronounced congenital proptosis (1–5). The globe usually is pushed forward and upward by the mass, and there may be marked conjunctival chemosis and eyelid swelling. The tumor can extend to involve the temporal fossa and other adjacent orbital tissues. Most orbital teratomas are benign, and malignant transformation is extremely rare. The globe usually is not affected. Histopathologically, teratoma can contain dermal elements (dermoid cyst), mesenchymal elements (cartilage), and endodermal tissue (gut, pancreas). Management consists of performing imaging studies to ascertain the extent of the disease and undertaking well-planned surgical removal. In the past, it often was necessary to remove the eye, but it is advisable to attempt to save the eye when possible.

SELECTED REFERENCES

1. Shields JA. *Diagnosis and management of orbital tumors.* Philadelphia: WB Saunders, 1989:97–102.
2. Henderson JW. *Orbital tumors,* 3rd ed. New York: Raven Press, 1994:61–64.
3. Soares EJC, Lopes KDS, Andrade JDS, et al. Orbital malignant teratoma. A case report. *Orbit* 1983; 2:235–242.
4. Ferry AP. Teratoma of the orbit: a report of two cases. *Surv Ophthalmol* 1965;10:434–443.
5. Chang DF, Dallow RL, Walton DS. Congenital orbital teratoma: report of a case with visual preservation. *J Pediatr Ophthalmol Strabismus* 1980;17:33–35.

Teratoma

Fig. 2-50 courtesy of Dr. Eduardo Soares. From Soares EJC, Lopes KDS, Andrade JDS, et al. Orbital malignant teratoma. A case report. *Orbit* 1983;2:235–242.

Figs. 2-53 and 2-54 courtesy of Dr. David Walton. From Chang DF, Dallow RL, Walton DS. Congenital orbital teratoma: report of a case with visual preservation. *J Pediatr Ophthalmol Strabismus* 1980;17:33–35.

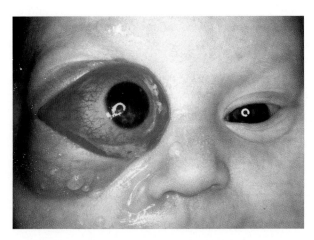

Figure 2-49. Orbital teratoma causing severe proptosis and chemosis in a baby girl. (Courtesy of Dr. Guy Allaire.)

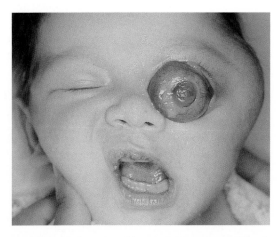

Figure 2-50. Malignant orbitocranial teratoma. The lesion affected the orbit, temporal fossa, and cranial cavity.

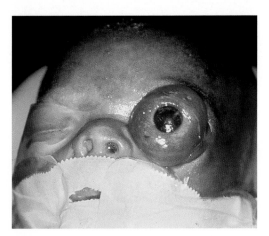

Figure 2-51. Orbital teratoma causing proptosis and chemosis in a newborn. (Courtesy of Dr. Lois Martyn.)

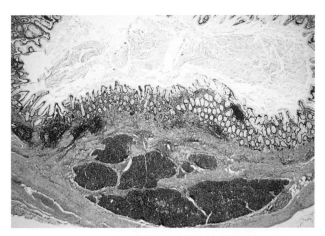

Figure 2-52. Histopathology of orbital teratoma showing intestinal mucosa and glandular tissue compatible with pancreas (hematoxylin–eosin, original magnification × 10). (Courtesy of Dr. Andrew Ferry and Armed Forces Institute of Pathology, Washington, DC.)

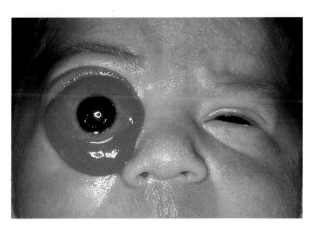

Figure 2-53. Newborn child with marked proptosis and chemosis secondary to orbital teratoma.

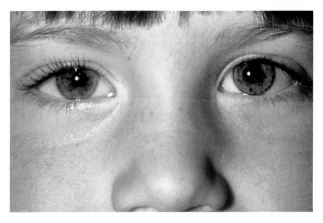

Figure 2-54. Appearance of the child shown in Fig. 2-53 several years later. The retrobulbar tumor was removed successfully and the eye was saved.

CONGENITAL CYSTIC EYE

Congenital cystic eye is an cystic orbital mass that results from a failure in the invagination of the primary optic vesicle between the 2- and 7-mm stage of fetal development. It can occur in an otherwise normal child, or it can be associated with other developmental abnormalities, such as cleft lip and palate, holoprosencephaly, and various other congenital lesions. Imaging studies reveal a large orbital cyst without evidence of a normal eye. The lesion consists of primitive neuroectodermal tissue, immature lens, and other primitive ocular structures (1–3).

SELECTED REFERENCES

1. Shields JA. *Diagnosis and management of orbital tumors.* Philadelphia: WB Saunders, 1989:102–104.
2. Henderson JW. *Orbital tumors*, 3rd ed. New York: Raven Press, 1994:67–68.
3. Mansour AM, Li HK. Congenital cystic eye. *Ophthal Plast Reconstr Surg* 1996;12:104–105.

Congenital Cystic Eye

Figs. 2-57 through 2-60 courtesy of Dr Ahmad Mansour. From Mansour AM, Li HK. Congenital cystic eye. *Ophthal Plast Reconstr Surg* 1996;12:104–105.

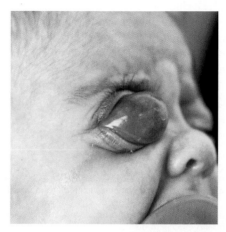

Figure 2-55. Soft-tissue mass protruding through the palpebral aperture in a infant girl. (Courtesy of Dr. Charles Specht.)

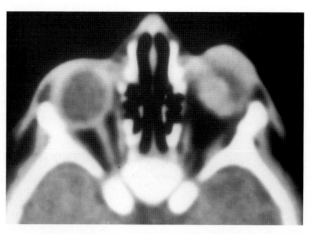

Figure 2-56. Axial computed tomogram of the patient shown in Fig. 2-55 depicting an irregular radiodensity in the right orbit with cystic features. The mass was removed and congenital cystic eye was documented. (Courtesy of Dr. Charles Specht.)

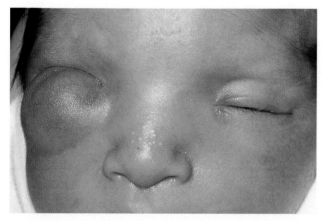

Figure 2-57. Blue-colored cystic mass deep to the right lower eyelid in an infant girl who also had holoprosencephaly, tetralogy of Fallot, low-set ears, webbed neck, and other systemic abnormalities.

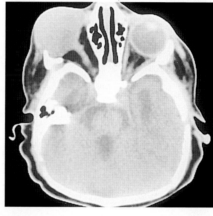

Figure 2-58. Axial computed tomogram of the patient shown in Fig. 2-57 showing cystic mass filling the orbit with a rudimentary optic nerve.

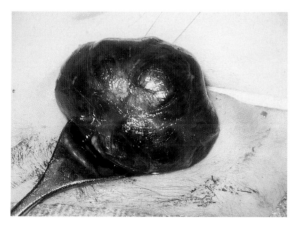

Figure 2-59. Surgical view of the lesion shown in Fig. 2-57 showing multilobular blue mass being removed after dissection from the adjacent periosteum.

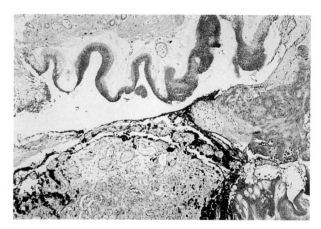

Figure 2-60. Histopathology of a portion of the lesion shown in Fig. 2-59 revealing a cleavage plane between (hematoxylin–eosin, original magnification × 40).

COLOBOMATOUS CYST

Colobomatous cyst (microphthalmos with cyst) is a congenital abnormality that consists of a small malformed eye with a coloboma through which a cystic herniation of glial tissue protrudes into the orbit (1,2). Because most colobomas are located inferonasally, the cyst usually causes protrusion of the lower eyelid beneath the small eye. In some cases, the cyst is not recognized clinically but is seen on computed tomography or magnetic resonance imaging as a cystic lesion inferior and posterior to a small eye (3). Pathologically, there is a small, often malformed, eye with a cyst attached inferonasally. It is lined by neuroectodermal tissue, and the cyst and the eyeball may exhibit massive gliosis (4). Treatment is surgical removal of the eye and the attached cyst if it causes significant symptoms (1,2).

SELECTED REFERENCES

1. Shields JA. *Diagnosis and management of orbital tumors.* Philadelphia: WB Saunders, 1989:104.
2. Waring GO II, Roth AM, Rodrigues MM. Clinicopathologic correlation of microphthalmos with cyst. *Am J Ophthalmol* 1976;82:714–721.
3. Weiss A, Greenwald M, Martinez C. Microphthalmos with cyst: clinical presentations and computed tomographic findings. *J Pediatr Ophthalmol Strabismus* 1985;22:6–12.
4. Nowinski T, Shields JA, Augsburger JJ, Devenuto JJ. Exophthalmos secondary to massive intraocular gliosis in a patient with a colobomatous cyst. *Am J Ophthalmol* 1984;97:641–643.

Colobomatous Cyst

Figs. 2-63 and 2-64 courtesy of Dr. Avery Weiss. From Weiss A, Greenwald M, Martinez C. Microphthalmos with cyst: clinical presentations and computed tomographic findings. *J Pediatr Ophthalmol Strabismus* 1985;22:6–12.

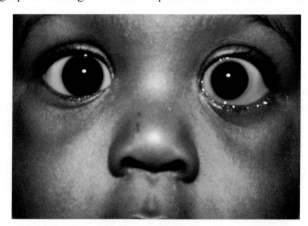

Figure 2-61. Microphthalmia of the left eye in a young child. (Courtesy of Dr. William Dickerson.)

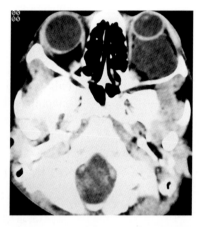

Figure 2-62. Axial computed tomogram of the patient shown in Fig. 2-61 demonstrating a small eye with a large retrobulbar cyst. (Courtesy of Dr. William Dickerson.)

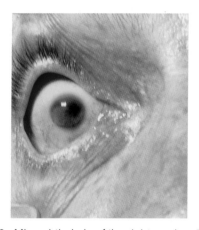

Figure 2-63. Microphthalmia of the right eye in a 57-year-old man.

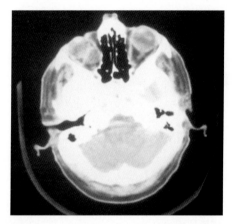

Figure 2-64. Axial computed tomogram of the patient shown in Fig. 2-63 revealing a cystic lesion posterior to the microphthalmic eye.

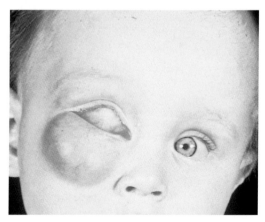

Figure 2-65. Typical appearance of colobomatous cyst with upward displacement of the microphthalmic eye and protrusion of the lower eyelid secondary to a large inferior orbital cyst. (Courtesy of Dr. Lorenz Zimmerman and Armed Forces Institute of Pathology, Washington, DC.)

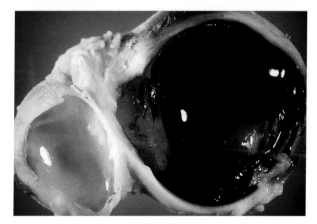

Figure 2-66. Gross appearance of microphthalmic eye and colobomatous cyst. (Courtesy of Dr. Lorenz Zimmerman and Armed Forces Institute of Pathology, Washington, DC.)

MENINGOCELE AND MENINGOENCEPHALOCELE

Congenital or acquired defects in the orbital bones may be associated protrusion of meningeal or brain tissue into the orbit. Meningoencephalocele of orbit can be divided into anterior and posterior types. The anterior (ethmoidal) type characteristically appears as a smooth subcutaneous fluctuant mass on the side of the nose near the medial canthus. It occasionally is bilateral. The posterior (sphenoidal) type protrudes into the orbit through the superior orbital fissure or the optic foramen (1). A characteristic feature is rhythmic pulsating proptosis. In some cases, the brain tissue may lose its connection to the cranial cavity and occur as ectopic brain tissue in the orbit (1–3). Other ocular abnormalities that may be associated with meningoencephalocele include anophthalmia, microphthalmia, cryptophthalmia, coloboma, and dysplastic optic disc. Treatment generally is surgical excision, which often requires a joint approach with an ophthalmologist, otolaryngologist, and neurosurgeon.

SELECTED REFERENCES

1. Shields JA. *Diagnosis and management of orbital tumors.* Philadelphia: WB Saunders, 1989:105–109.
2. Henderson JW. *Orbital tumors,* 3rd ed. New York: Raven Press, 1994:64–66.
3. Newman NJ, Miller NR, Green WR. Ectopic brain in the orbit. *Ophthalmology* 1986;93:268–272.

Meningocele and Meningoencephalocele

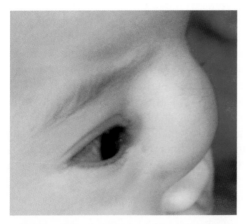

Figure 2-67. Anterior meningoencephalocele in an infant showing the smooth subcutaneous mass in the region of the medial canthus.

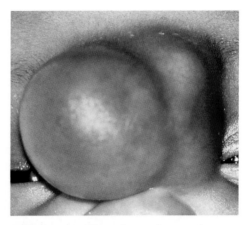

Figure 2-68. Larger bilateral anterior meningoencephalocele over the nasal area in an infant. (Courtesy of Dr. Darrell Wolfley.)

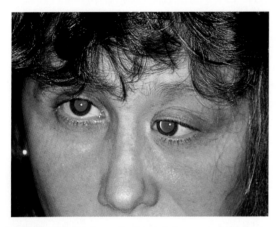

Figure 2-69. Marked proptosis and downward displacement of the left eye secondary to a posterior orbital meningoencephalocele in a 37-year-old woman who had neurofibromatosis and absence of the sphenoid wing.

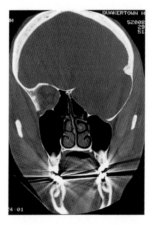

Figure 2-70. Coronal computed tomogram of the patient shown in Fig. 2-69 demonstrating marked herniation of brain into the posterior orbit through the area of bony absence.

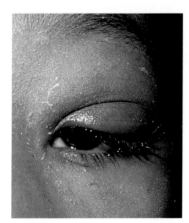

Figure 2-71. Child with slight proptosis, blepharoptosis, and upper eyelid edema of the left eye secondary to posterior orbital meningoencephalocele.

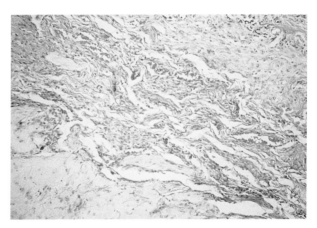

Figure 2-72. Histopathology of meningoencephalocele showing mature brain and meningeal tissue.

MUCOCELE

A mucocele is a cystic lesion that contains mucous. If a mucocele becomes secondarily infected, it is called a mucopyocele. Most mucoceles that affect the orbit arise from the frontal or ethmoid sinuses and secondarily involve the orbit (1). It usually develops in adults with chronic sinusitis, but it can occur in children, particularly in patients with cystic fibrosis. Mucocele accounted for 2% of all biopsied orbital masses and for 8% of all biopsied orbital cystic lesions in the authors' series (2). The patient usually has a history of chronic sinusitis and presents with fluctuant superonasal orbital mass (3,4). Imaging studies demonstrate cloudy sinuses and a cystic mass eroding through the bone into the orbit (5). Histopathologically, there is a cystic lesion lined by sinus respiratory epithelium with inflammation in the adjacent tissues. The management is surgical excision, culture and sensitivity, and drainage of the lesion.

SELECTED REFERENCES

1. Shields JA. *Diagnosis and management of orbital tumors.* Philadelphia: WB Saunders, 1989:113–115.
2. Shields JA, Bakewell B, Augsburger DG, Flanagan CJ. Classification and incidence of space-occupying lesions of the orbit. A survey of 645 biopsies. *Arch Ophthalmol* 1984;102:1606–1611.
3. Iliff CE. Mucoceles in the orbit. *Arch Ophthalmol* 1973;89:392–395.
4. Avery G, Tang RA, Close LG. Ophthalmic manifestations of mucoceles. *Ann Ophthalmol* 1983;15:734–737.
5. Valvassori GE, Putterman AM. Ophthalmological and radiological findings in sphenoidal mucoceles. *Arch Ophthalmol* 1973;90:456–459.

Mucocele

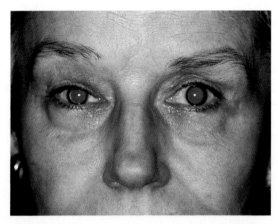

Figure 2-73. Downward and temporal displacement of the right eye in 66-year-old woman.

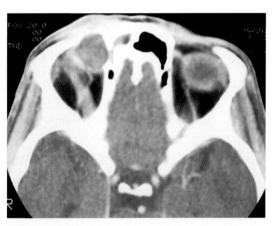

Figure 2-74. Axial computed tomogram of the patient shown in Fig. 2-73. Note the cloudy sinus and the cystic structure in the superonasal portion of the orbit.

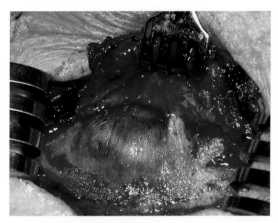

Figure 2-75. Mucocele in the patient shown in Fig. 2-73 as seen at the time of surgical exposure. The adherent cyst was aspirated and the sinus was exenterated with removal of its epithelium.

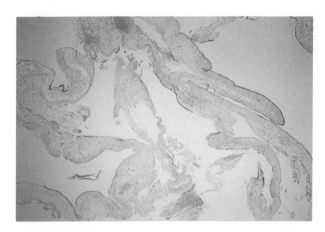

Figure 2-76. Histopathology of the lesion shown in Fig. 2-75. Note the collapsed cystic structure with sinus epithelium and chronic inflammation in the walls (hematoxylin–eosin, original magnification × 10).

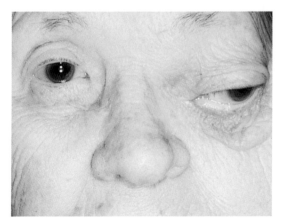

Figure 2-77. Inferotemporal displacement of the left eye in an 84-year-old woman with a long history of proptosis. (Courtesy of Dr. John Bullock.)

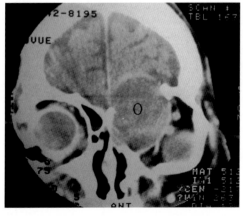

Figure 2-78. Coronal computed tomogram of the patient shown in Fig. 2-77 showing a 4-cm cystic mass with bony destruction. (Courtesy of Dr. John Bullock.)

RESPIRATORY CYST

Mucoceles are lined by sinus respiratory epithelium. However, there are other types of cysts lined by respiratory epithelium that can occur in the orbit. Choristomatous respiratory cyst can occur as a congenital orbital cystic lesion. An acquired respiratory cyst can be idiopathic (perhaps congenital and previously unrecognized) or it can occur following trauma. It differs from a mucocele in that the affected patient does not have sinusitis and may not display severe inflammation (1–3). Because the diagnosis usually is not made clinically, most symptomatic lesions are excised, which is the treatment of choice.

SELECTED REFERENCES

1. Shields JA. *Diagnosis and management of orbital tumors.* Philadelphia: WB Saunders, 1989:113–115.
2. Newton C, Dutton JJ, Klintworth GK. A respiratory epithelial choristomatous cyst of the orbit. *Ophthalmology* 1985;9:1754–1757.
3. James CRH, Lyness R, Wright JE. Respiratory epithelium lined cysts presenting in the orbit without associated mucocele formation. *Br J Ophthalmol* 1986;70:387–390.

Respiratory Cyst

Figs. 2-79 through 2-81 courtesy of Dr. Jonathan Dutton. From Newton C, Dutton JJ, Klintworth GK. A respiratory epithelial choristomatous cyst of the orbit. *Ophthalmology* 1985;9:1754–1757.

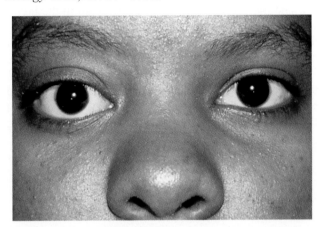

Figure 2-79. Proptosis of the right eye in a 23-year-old woman. It was noted at age 4 years, had been slowly progressive, and had produced intermittent episodes of pain.

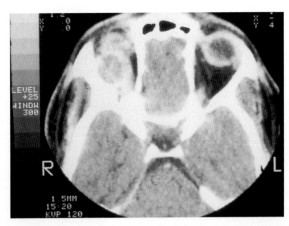

Figure 2-80. Axial computed tomogram of the patient shown in Fig. 2-79 revealing a cystic lesion producing anterior and downward displacement of the right eye.

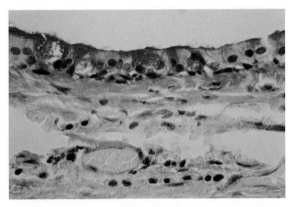

Figure 2-81. Histopathology of the lesion shown in Fig. 2-80 demonstrating the respiratory epithelium with goblet cells (hematoxylin–eosin, original magnification × 200).

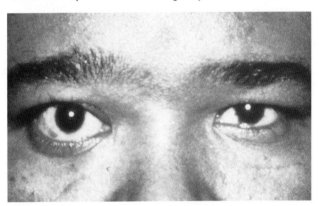

Figure 2-82. Proptosis of the right eye in a 37-year-old man. Proptosis had been present for most of his life, but it had recently become progressively worse. (Courtesy of Dr. William R. Morris.)

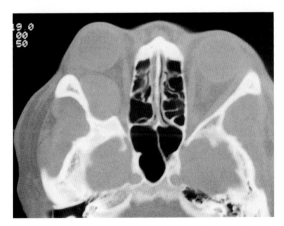

Figure 2-83. Axial computed tomogram of the patient shown in Fig. 2-82 revealing a homogeneous mass causing proptosis of the right eye. The lesion was excised. (Courtesy of Dr. William R. Morris.)

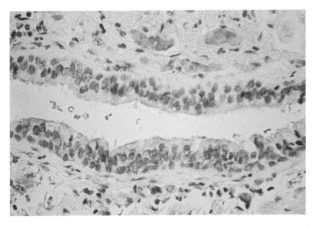

Figure 2-84. Histopathology of the lesion shown in Fig. 2-83 demonstrating the ciliated respiratory epithelium that lined the mass (hematoxylin–eosin, original magnification × 200). (Courtesy of Dr. William R. Morris.)

PARASITIC CYSTS—HYDATID CYST

A number of parasitic infestations can affect the orbit and produce an orbital cyst that contains the parasite (1). Hydatid cyst is the infestation of tissue by the larva of tapeworm of the genus *Echinococcus*. The definitive host is the dog, and humans can be involved as accidental hosts. The life cycle is reported in more detail in the literature (1). Although rare in North America, it is a common cause of proptosis, particularly in teenagers, in Africa, the Middle East, and South America. The infected patient presents with progressive proptosis, ocular pain, oculomotor palsies, optic disc edema, and sometimes optic atrophy. Systemic evaluation usually fails to reveal other sites of *Echinococcus* infection. Management is surgical removal, which may require a lateral orbitotomy for deeply located lesions (2). Cysticercosis also can occur in the orbit (3,4). It is the infestation of tissue by *Cysticercus cellulosae*, the larval form of the pig tapeworm, *Taenia solium*.

SELECTED REFERENCES

1. Shields JA. *Diagnosis and management of orbital tumors.* Philadelphia: WB Saunders, 1989:113–115.
2. Gomez Morales A, Croxatto JO, Crovetto L, Ebner R. Hydatid cysts of the orbit. A review of 35 cases. *Ophthalmology* 1988;95:1027–1032.
3. Sekhar GC, Lemke BN. Orbital cysticercosis. *Ophthalmology* 1978;104:2599-2604.
4. Bonavolonta G, Tranfa F. An unusual orbital cyst. *Orbit* 1984;3:179–182.

Hydatid Cyst

Figs. 2-87 through 2-90 courtesy of Dr. Giulio Bonavolonta. From Bonavolonta G, Tranfa F. An unusual orbital cyst. *Orbit* 1984;3:179–182.

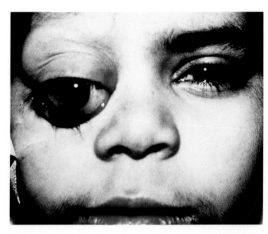

Figure 2-85. Proptosis and downward displacement of the right eye secondary to orbital hydatid cyst in a 6-year-old girl. There was 17 mm of proptosis, total impairment of ocular motility, and vision of finger counting in the affected right eye. (Courtesy of Dr. J. Oscar Croxatto.)

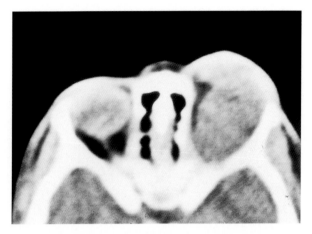

Figure 2-86. Axial computed tomogram of the patient shown in Fig. 2-85 demonstrating a large cystic mass in the orbit causing marked proptosis and displacement of the globe. (Courtesy of Dr. J. Oscar Croxatto.)

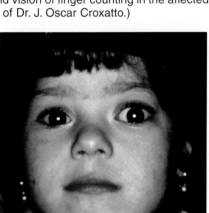

Figure 2-87. Proptosis of the left eye in a 4-year-old girl.

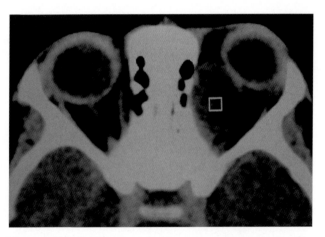

Figure 2-88. Orbital computed tomogram demonstrating the cystic mass in the orbit (marked with a *square*).

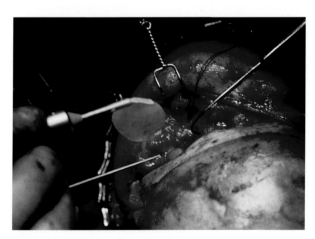

Figure 2-89. After surgical exposure, the cyst is being removed with a cryoprobe.

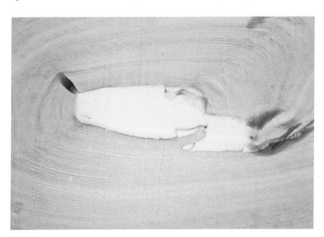

Figure 2-90. Histopathology of the lesion shown in Fig. 2-89 demonstrating the capsule of the cyst composed of acellular hyaline material (hematoxylin–eosin, original magnification × 250).

CHAPTER 3

Vascular and Hemorrhagic Lesions

CAPILLARY HEMANGIOMA

Capillary hemangioma (benign hemangioendothelioma, strawberry hemangioma) is an important cutaneous vascular tumor of childhood. It can also occur in the orbit (1). In the authors' series, it accounted for 1% of all biopsied orbital lesions in all age groups (2) and for 4% of all orbital biopsies in children (3). The subject of its occurrence on the eyelid is discussed in the *Atlas of Eyelid and Conjunctival Tumors*. When it occurs in the orbit, it generally is apparent shortly after birth as a fluctuant mass deep to the eyelid (1,4). Occasionally, it develops in the deeper portions of the orbit without eyelid signs. Extension of the lesion on the periocular skin facilitates diagnosis. The main complications are amblyopia and strabismus. The lesion usually shows gradual enlargement for 1 to 2 years and then undergoes gradual regression. Imaging studies show an irregular or diffuse mass that enhances with contrast material. Orbital capillary hemangioma may be associated with large visceral hemangiomas that can cause platelet entrapment and thrombocytopenia, a condition called the Kasabach–Merritt syndrome (1). Histopathologically, it is composed of lobules of proliferating endothelial cells separated by thin fibrous tissue septa. Initial management should include refraction and occlusive treatment of associated amblyopia. If there is no threat to vision, the lesion can be observed cautiously. Oral or local injection of corticosteroids may hasten regression of the lesion, but corticosteroids have a number of potential complications. Surgical excision is an appropriate treatment for selected well-circumscribed tumors (5).

SELECTED REFERENCES

1. Shields JA. *Diagnosis and management of orbital tumors*. Philadelphia: WB Saunders, 1989:124–128.
2. Shields JA, Bakewell B, Augsburger DG, Flanagan JC. Classification and incidence of space-occupying lesions of the orbit. A survey of 645 biopsies. *Arch Ophthalmol* 1984;102:1606–1611.
3. Shields JA, Bakewell B, Augsburger DG, Donoso LA, Bernardino V. Space-occupying orbital masses in children. A review of 250 consecutive biopsies. *Ophthalmology* 1986;93:379–384.
4. Haik BG, Jakobiec FA, Ellsworth RM, Jones IS. Capillary hemangioma of the lids and orbit: an analysis of the clinical features and therapeutic results in 101 cases. *Ophthalmology* 1979;86:760–792.
5. Deans RM, Harris GJ, Kivlin JD. Surgical dissection of capillary hemangiomas. An alternative to intralesional corticosteroids. *Arch Ophthalmol* 1992;110:1743–1747.

Orbital Capillary Hemangioma—Clinical Variations

Orbital capillary hemangioma can occur in the deep orbit and produce proptosis or displacement of the globe, or it can occur in the anterior portion of the orbit and present as a reddish-blue, fluctuant subcutaneous eyelid mass.

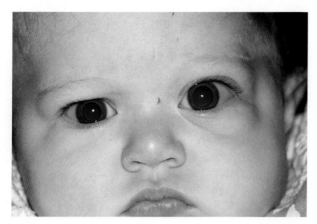

Figure 3-1. Prominence of the left lower eyelid secondary to orbital capillary hemangioma in a 4-month-old girl.

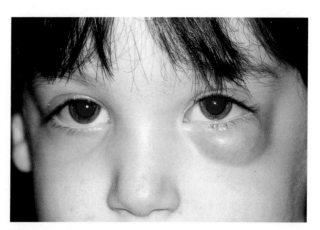

Figure 3-2. Prominence of the left lower eyelid secondary to orbital capillary hemangioma in a 2-year-old girl.

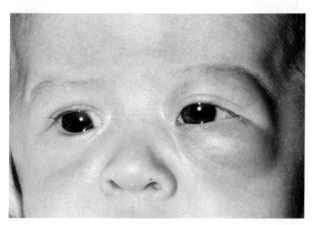

Figure 3-3. Prominence of the left lower and upper eyelid secondary to orbital capillary hemangioma in a 1-year-old girl.

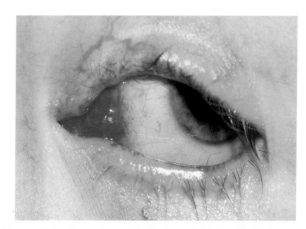

Figure 3-4. Extension of orbital capillary hemangioma into the medial aspect of the conjunctiva. The child had visceral hemangiomas and may have had a variant of the Kasabach–Merritt syndrome.

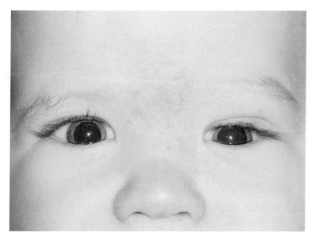

Figure 3-5. Slight downward displacement of the left eye in an 8-month-old boy with orbital capillary hemangioma.

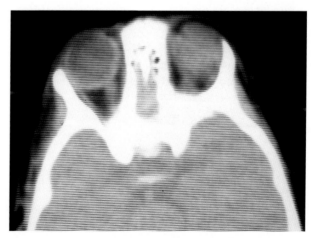

Figure 3-6. Axial computed tomogram of the child shown in Fig. 3-5 demonstrating a diffuse mass superior to the left eye..

Orbital Capillary Hemangioma—Clinical Variations and Regression

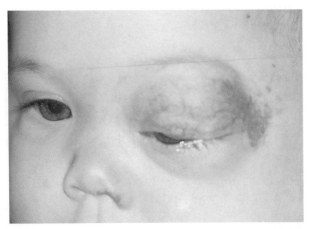

Figure 3-7. Proptosis of the left eye in a 4-month-old girl. The associated cutaneous hemangioma should suggest an orbital hemangioma as the cause of the proptosis.

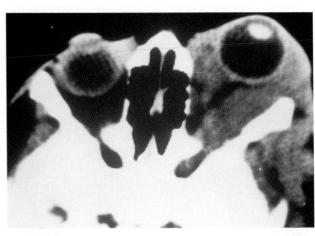

Figure 3-8. Axial computed tomogram of the patient shown in Fig. 3-7. Note the diffuse involvement of the orbital soft tissues.

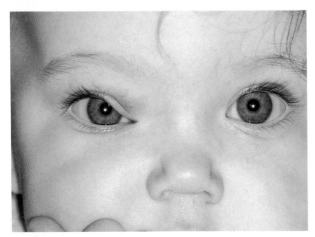

Figure 3-9. Characteristic subcutaneous mass superonasal to the right eye in a 5-month-old girl.

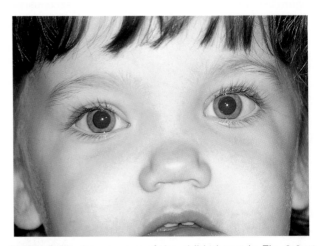

Figure 3-10. Appearance of the child shown in Fig. 3-9 at age 23 months. The lesion has shown regression without treatment.

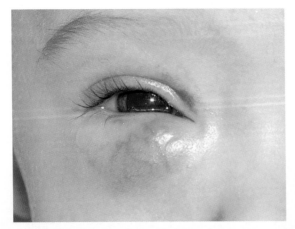

Figure 3-11. Reddish-blue subcutaneous mass beneath the right lower eyelid in a 4-month-old boy.

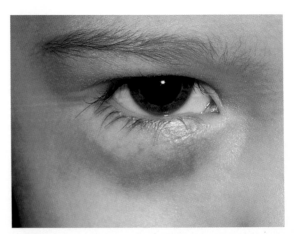

Figure 3-12. Appearance of the child shown in Fig. 3-11 at age 24 months. The lesion has shown regression without treatment.

Orbital Capillary Hemangioma—Surgical Resection

Surgical excision may be the best treatment of large, anterior, well-circumscribed orbital capillary hemangiomas that are producing significant ocular signs and symptoms. A clinicopathologic correlation is shown.

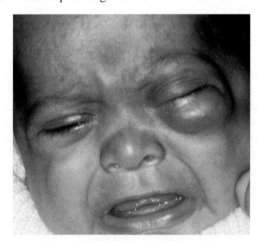

Figure 3-13. Extensive inferior orbital mass producing a prominent blue appearance to the left lower eyelid in an infant girl.

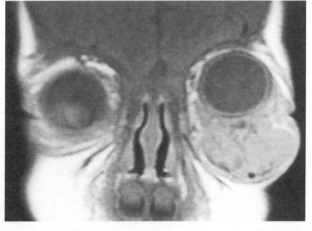

Figure 3-14. Coronal magnetic resonance imaging in T1-weighted image, showing large but fairly well-circumscribed inferior orbital mass. The mass was removed via an eyelid incision.

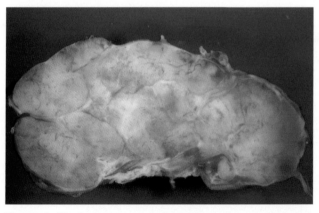

Figure 3-15. Appearance of the lesion after surgical excision and fixation showing that the lesion was removed intact.

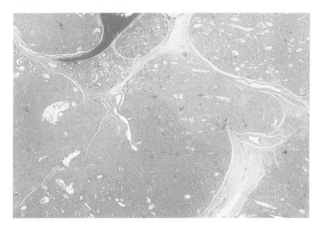

Figure 3-16. Low-magnification photomicrograph showing the vascular lobules with connective tissue septa (hematoxylin–eosin, original magnification × 20).

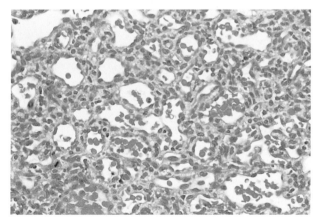

Figure 3-17. Histopathology of the lesion showing proliferation of small vascular channels (hematoxylin–eosin, original magnification × 150).

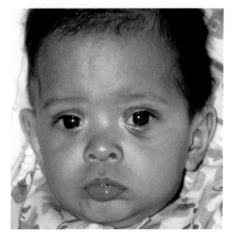

Figure 3-18. Appearance of the same child 7 weeks after surgery.

CAVERNOUS HEMANGIOMA

Cavernous hemangioma is the most common vascular tumor of the orbit (1–5). It is a benign tumor that tends to occur in adulthood as a relatively stationary or slowly progressive lesion that can produce painless proptosis (1–5). Because it most often occurs in the muscle cone, it usually produces axial proptosis. It generally does not produce inflammatory signs. Since the advent of good imaging techniques such as computed tomography and magnetic resonance imaging, this tumor often is being discovered as a coincidental finding when it is small and asymptomatic. As it slowly enlarges, it can produce marked proptosis, compression of the optic nerve, and choroidal folds. Imaging studies demonstrate a well-circumscribed, round to oval mass, usually in the muscle cone. It shows mild enhancement with contrast agents. The differential diagnosis of a well-circumscribed, round to ovoid, solid orbital mass also includes neurilemoma, hemangiopericytoma, fibrous histiocytoma, melanoma, and several other orbital tumors. It occasionally can be bilateral or multiple in one orbit, and it sometimes can be located within bone (6). Histopathologically, it is composed of dilated, congested vascular channels separated by connective tissue that contains smooth muscle. Management ranges from periodic observation for small asymptomatic lesions to surgical excision for larger symptomatic tumors. The surgical approach is determined by the size and location of the tumor. A conjunctival approach or cutaneous approach may be used for anterior lesions. Deep orbital tumors may require a lateral orbitotomy, sometimes with an osteotomy (Kronlein approach). Complete excision is important, and the surgery should be done by skilled orbital surgeons to avoid incomplete excision and recurrence.

SELECTED REFERENCES

1. Shields JA. *Diagnosis and management of orbital tumors.* Philadelphia: WB Saunders, 1989:128–132.
2. Shields JA, Bakewell B, Augsburger DG, Flanagan CJ. Classification and incidence of space-occupying lesions of the orbit. A survey of 645 biopsies. *Arch Ophthalmol* 1984;102:1606–1611.
3. Rootman J, Graeb A. Vascular lesions. Cavernous hemangiomas. In: Rootman J, ed. *Diseases of the orbit.* Philadelphia: JB Lippincott Co., 1988:532–533.
4. Henderson JW. *Orbital tumors,* 3rd ed. New York: Raven Press, 1994:95–100.
5. Harris GJ, Jakobiec FA. Cavernous hemangioma of the orbit: a clinicopathologic analysis of sixty-six cases. In: Jakobiec FA, ed: *Ocular and adnexal tumors.* Birmingham: Aesculapius Publishing Co., 1978:741–781.
6. Hornblass A, Zaidman GW. Intraosseous orbital cavernous hemangioma. *Ophthalmology* 1981;88:1351–1355.

Orbital Cavernous Hemangioma

With the advent of computed tomography and magnetic resonance imaging, some orbital cavernous hemangiomas are discovered at an early stage when they are asymptomatic. Such lesions generally are followed without treatment, because in some cases they may not become symptomatic for many years. Like other orbital tumors, they can produce fundus changes such as choroidal folds, optic disc edema, and compression of the globe. Examples are cited.

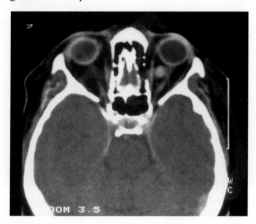

Figure 3-19. Axial computed tomogram of small asymptomatic cavernous hemangioma in the anterior orbit immediately posterior to the globe.

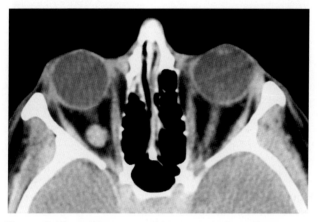

Figure 3-20. Axial computed tomogram of small asymptomatic cavernous hemangioma closer to the orbital apex.

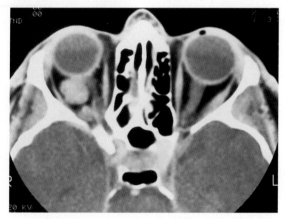

Figure 3-21. Axial computed tomogram of slightly larger but asymptomatic cavernous hemangioma in midportion of the orbit in muscle cone.

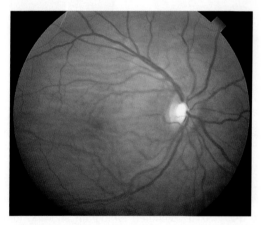

Figure 3-22. Fundus photograph showing characteristic horizontal choroidal folds secondary to an intraconal cavernous hemangioma.

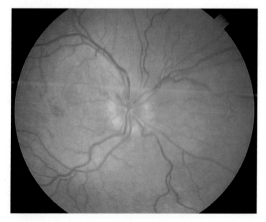

Figure 3-23. Optic disc edema secondary to optic nerve compression of orbital cavernous hemangioma.

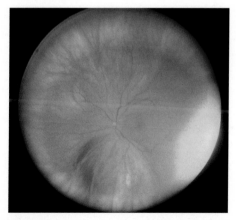

Figure 3-24. Wide-angle fundus photograph showing compression of inferior portion of the globe by an orbital cavernous hemangioma. Such an elevation sometimes can be confused with an intraocular neoplasm.

Orbital Cavernous Hemangioma Removed Through a Conjunctival Incision

A clinicopathologic correlation of a tumor removed through a horizontal forniceal conjunctiva is depicted.

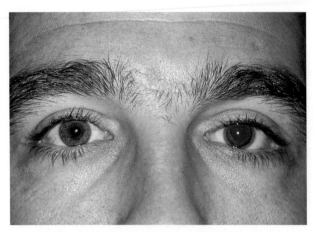

Figure 3-25. Slight proptosis of the left eye in a 40-year-old man. The pupil was dilated from mydriatic drops.

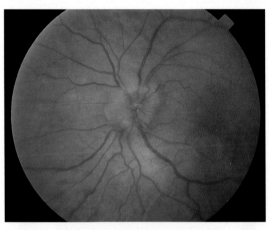

Figure 3-26. Optic disc edema secondary to optic nerve compression by the tumor.

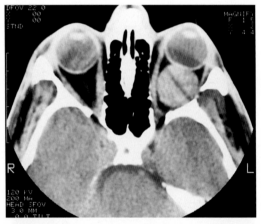

Figure 3-27. Axial computed tomogram showing tumor in the muscle cone.

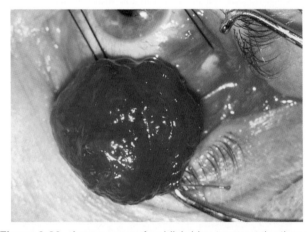

Figure 3-28. Appearance of reddish-blue tumor at the time of removal via a conjunctival incision.

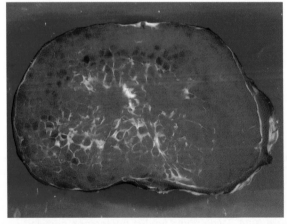

Figure 3-29. Gross appearance after sectioning showing red vascular tumor.

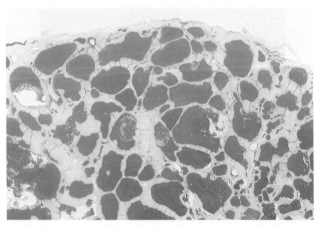

Figure 3-30. Histopathology showing the large congested cavernous vascular channels (hematoxylin–eosin, original magnification × 20).

Orbital Cavernous Hemangioma Removed Through a Superolateral Orbitotomy

Larger tumors in the muscle cone or tumors located laterally in the posterior aspect of the orbit are best approached by a superolateral orbitotomy with a skin incision. An osteotomy (Kronlein approach) usually is not necessary.

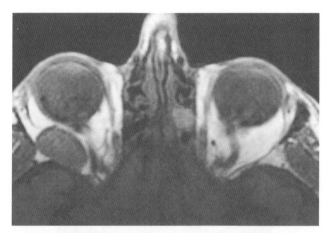

Figure 3-31. Axial magnetic resonance imaging in T1-weighted image showing circumscribed mass in posterolateral aspect of the orbit in a 66-year-old man.

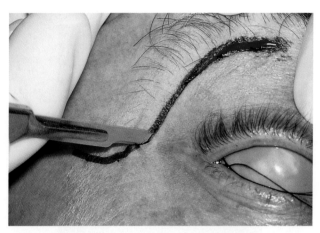

Figure 3-32. Outline of superolateral orbitotomy by a classic cutaneous incision in the patient shown in Fig. 3-31.

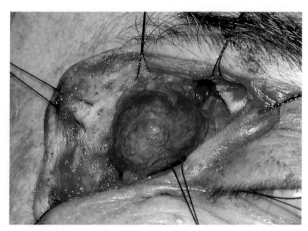

Figure 3-33. Same tumor being removed without an osteotomy.

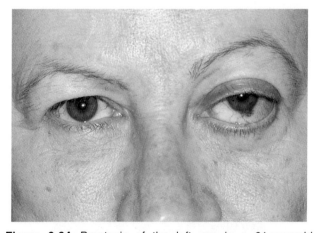

Figure 3-34. Proptosis of the left eye in a 61-year-old woman.

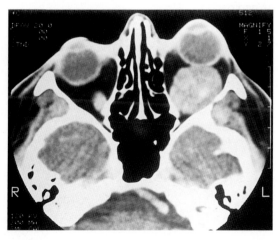

Figure 3-35. Axial computed tomogram of the woman shown in Fig. 3-34 demonstrating a large mass in the muscle cone extending almost to the orbital apex.

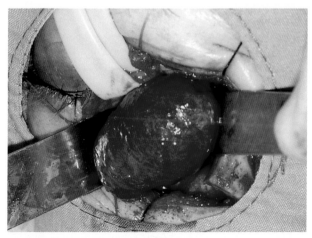

Figure 3-36. Tumor shown in Fig. 3-35 being removed by superolateral orbitotomy with osteotomy.

Orbital Cavernous Hemangioma Removed Through a Superomedial Orbitotomy

In cases where the tumor is nasal to the optic nerve, a superomedial orbitotomy can be employed. Although a conjunctival incision could have been used in the case shown, the skin–extraperiosteal approach offers better surgical exposure.

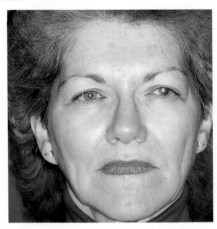

Figure 3-37. Proptosis of the left eye in a 52-year-old woman. The patient was followed for 5 years previously, during which proptosis increased and optic disc compression occurred. The pupil was dilated due to mydriatic drops.

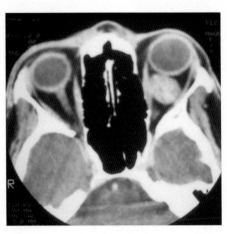

Figure 3-38. Axial computed tomogram showing a mass in the muscle cone.

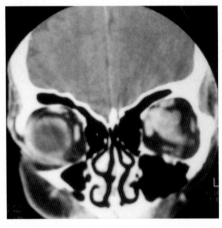

Figure 3-39. Coronal computed tomogram showing that the mass is nasal to the optic nerve.

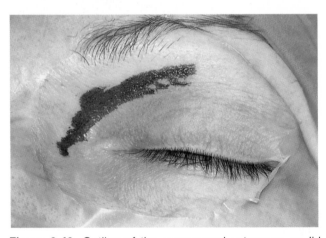

Figure 3-40. Outline of the superonasal cutaneous eyelid crease approach.

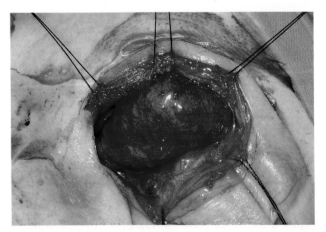

Figure 3-41. Tumor exposed via a superonasal approach.

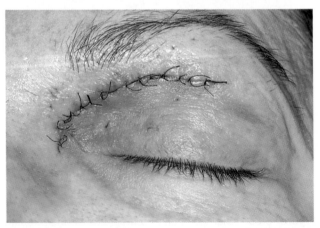

Figure 3-42. Appearance of the wound after closure with interrupted 6-0 silk sutures.

Intraosseous Orbital Cavernous Hemangioma

In rare instances, a cavernous hemangioma can occur in the bone, rather than being confined to the orbital soft tissues.

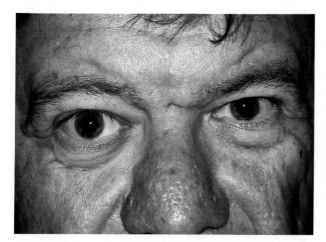

Figure 3-43. Proptosis of the right eye in a 57-year-old man.

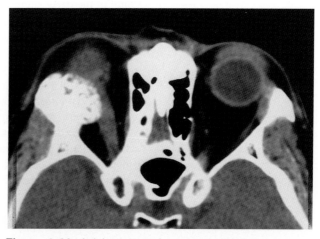

Figure 3-44. Axial computed tomogram showing a mass within bone on the lateral aspect of the orbit.

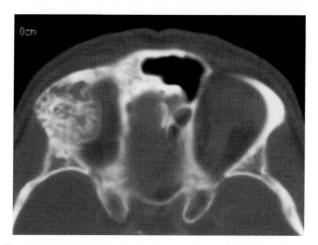

Figure 3-45. Axial computed tomogram using bone window technique showing the lesion.

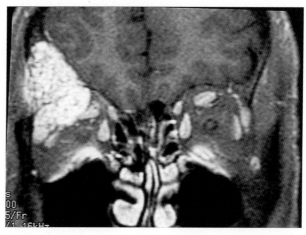

Figure 3-46. Coronal magnetic resonance imaging in T1-weighted image showing superior extent of the lesion in the frontal bone.

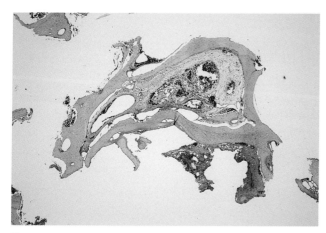

Figure 3-47. Histopathology of intraosseous cavernous hemangioma showing vascular mass in the bone (hematoxylin–eosin, original magnification × 5).

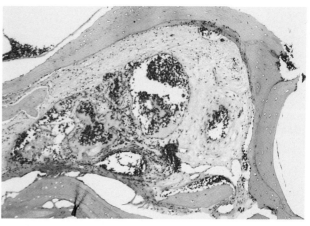

Figure 3-48. Slightly higher-power photomicrograph showing cavernous vascular channels (hematoxylin–eosin, original magnification × 15).

HEMANGIOPERICYTOMA

Hemangiopericytoma is a tumor composed of an abnormal proliferation of pericytes that surround blood vessels. It accounted for 1% of all orbital biopsies and 18% of all biopsies of vascular tumors in the authors' series (1,2). It occurs mainly in adults and in the early stages produces similar symptoms, signs, and imaging study findings as the cavernous hemangioma just described. With time, however, hemangiopericytoma can assume a more aggressive behavior pattern and violate its capsule, demonstrate florid growth in the orbit, and invade the cranial cavity (3–6). About 30% of orbital hemangiopericytomas have histopathologic criteria compatible with malignancy, but distant metastasis is rare (4). Because the diagnosis cannot be made with certainty of clinical evaluation, the management is the same as for other circumscribed primary tumors. A complete excision of the tumor in its capsule should be performed by an experienced orbital surgeon. The selected approach to surgery should depend on the results of good axial and coronal imaging studies. Orbital recurrence, which can develop many years after the original surgery, may require orbital exenteration, irradiation, or chemotherapy.

SELECTED REFERENCES

1. Shields JA. *Diagnosis and management of orbital tumors.* Philadelphia: WB Saunders, 1989:132–134.
2. Shields JA, Bakewell B, Augsberger JJ, Flanagan JC. Classification and incidence of space-occupying lesions of the orbit. A survey of 645 biopsies. *Arch Ophthalmol* 1984;102:1606–1111.
3. Henderson JW. *Orbital tumors,* 3rd ed. New York: Raven Press, 1994:95–100.
4. Croxatto JO, Font RL. Hemangiopericytoma of the orbit: a clinicopathologic study of 30 cases. *Hum Pathol* 1982;13:210–218.
5. Karcioglu ZA, Nasr AM, Haik BG. Orbital hemangiopericytoma: clinical and morphologic features. *Am J Ophthalmol* 1997;124;661–672.
6. Shields JA, Shields CL, Rashid RC. Clinicopathologic correlation of choroidal folds secondary to massive cranio-orbital hemangiopericytoma. *Ophthal Reconstr Plast Surg* 1992;8:62–68.

Hemangiopericytoma—Clinicopathologic Correlation

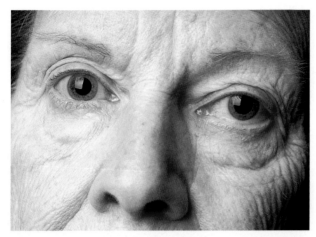

Figure 3-49. Proptosis of the left eye in a 72-year-old woman.

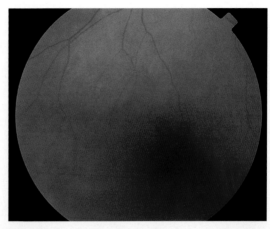

Figure 3-50. Fundus photograph showing compression of the globe inferiorly simulating a pigmented intraocular tumor.

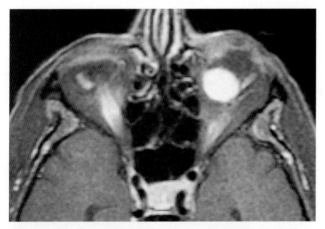

Figure 3-51. Contrast-enhanced axial magnetic resonance imaging demonstrating enhancing mass in the left orbit.

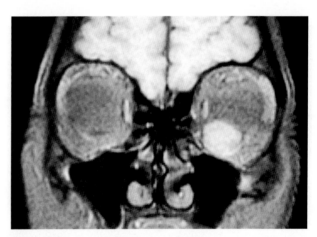

Figure 3-52. Coronal magnetic resonance imaging showing location of mass inferior to the globe.

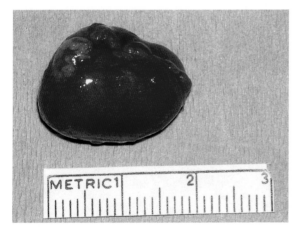

Figure 3-53. Circumscribed red tumor after surgical removal via a conjunctival approach.

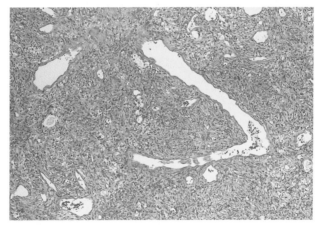

Figure 3-54. Histopathology showing solid vascular with typical "staghorn" branching of the blood vessels (hematoxylin–eosin, original magnification × 50).

Hemangiopericytoma—Clinicopathologic Correlation

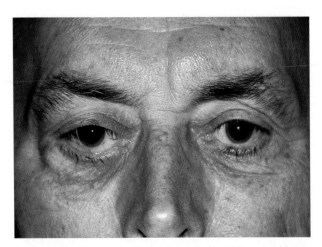

Figure 3-55. Proptosis of the right eye in a 63-year-old man.

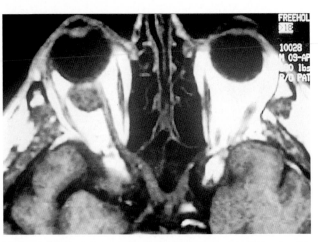

Figure 3-56. Axial magnetic resonance imaging in T1-weighted image showing retrobulbar mass that is compressing the globe.

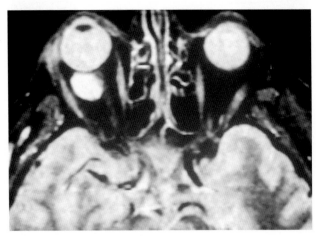

Figure 3-57. Axial magnetic resonance imaging in T2-weighted image showing retrobulbar mass that is hyperintense to the vitreous.

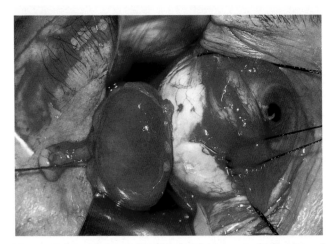

Figure 3-58. Appearance of the red circumscribed mass at the time of surgical removal via a conjunctival approach.

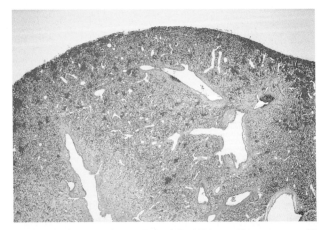

Figure 3-59. Histopathology showing solid tumor with "staghorn" branching pattern to the larger blood vessels (hematoxylin–eosin, original magnification × 25).

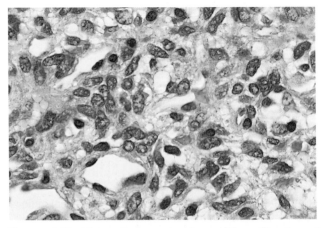

Figure 3-60. Histopathology showing solid proliferation of tumor cells (hematoxylin–eosin, original magnification × 200).

Aggressive Orbital Hemangiopericytoma with Invasion of Cranial Cavity

In some instances, hemangiopericytoma can undergo malignant transformation and can be locally invasive. Distant metastasis occasionally can develop. A clinicopathologic correlation is shown.

From Shields JA, Shields CL, Rashid RC. Clinicopathologic correlation of choroidal folds secondary to massive cranio-orbital hemangiopericytoma. *Ophthal Reconstr Plast Surg* 1992;8:62–68.

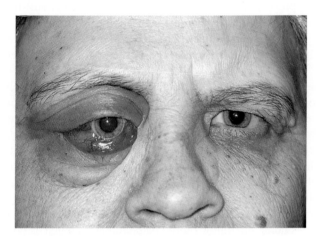

Figure 3-61. Marked proptosis and chemosis of the right eye in a 56-year-old woman.

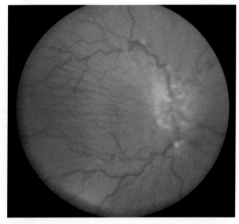

Figure 3-62. Fundus photograph showing optic disc edema and marked choroidal folds secondary to compression of the posterior aspect of the globe by the orbital tumor.

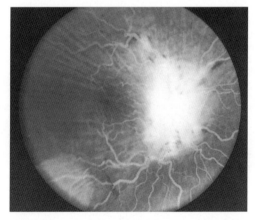

Figure 3-63. Fluorescein angiogram showing hyperfluorescence of the optic disc and radiating choroidal folds.

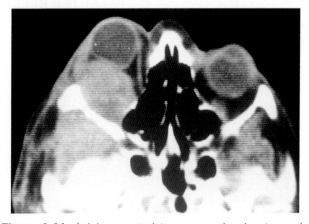

Figure 3-64. Axial computed tomogram showing tumor in the orbit and cranial cavity.

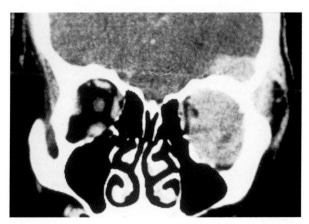

Figure 3-65. Coronal computed tomogram further delineating the extent of the tumor. It was removed by orbital exenteration and craniotomy.

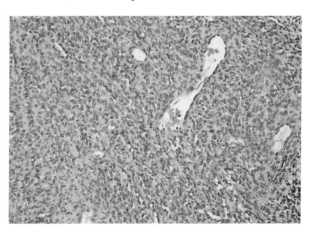

Figure 3-66. Histopathology showing characteristic pattern of hemangiopericytoma (hematoxylin–eosin, original magnification × 50).

LYMPHANGIOMA

Lymphangioma is a benign, slowly progressive tumor that probably is congenital but may not become clinically apparent for months or years after birth (1–6). In the authors' series of orbital tumors, it accounted for 1% of all orbital biopsies and 10% of all vasculogenic tumors (2). With the advent of good magnetic resonance imaging studies, it is being diagnosed more frequently. It usually has its clinical onset in children in the first few years of life. In many instances, it is not recognized until the teenage years, when the patient presents with abrupt proptosis and periocular soft-tissue swelling from spontaneous or traumatic hemorrhage in the lymphangioma. Affected patients may have lymphangiomas elsewhere, particularly on the palate. Imaging studies show a diffuse multiloculated mass with cystic spaces often filled with blood ("chocolate cysts").

Histopathologically, lymphangioma consists of dilated ectatic vascular channels filled with clear fluid or blood. Lymphoid cells frequently are present in the delicate connective tissue septa. Management can be a problem, because complete surgical resection is often difficult to impossible. If the visual acuity is not threatened in a young child, a period of observation, allowing the acute hemorrhage to resolve, is warranted (4,5). If massive tumor and hemorrhage cause unacceptable proptosis or optic nerve compression, then treatment should be considered. Large hemorrhagic cysts can be aspirated through the eyelid or conjunctiva to provide temporary relief. If malignancy, such as rhabdomyosarcoma, is a diagnostic possibility, exploration with open biopsy is warranted. If surgery is done, the tumor should be debulked as much as possible without damaging the optic nerve or extraocular muscles (1–7).

SELECTED REFERENCES

1. Shields JA. *Diagnosis and management of orbital tumors.* Philadelphia: WB Saunders, 1989:134–138.
2. Shields JA, Bakewell B, Augsberger JJ, Flanagan JC. Classification and incidence of space-occupying lesions of the orbit. A survey of 645 biopsies. *Arch Ophthalmol* 1984;102:1606–1611.
3. Rootman J, Hay E, Graeb D, Miller R. Orbital-adnexal lymphangiomas. A spectrum of hemodynamically isolated vascular hamartomas. *Ophthalmology* 1986;93:1558–1570.
4. Harris GJ, Sakol PJ, Bonavolonta G, de Conciliis C. An analysis of thirty cases of orbital lymphangioma. *Ophthalmology* 1990;97:1583–1592.
5. Wilson ME, Parker PL, Chavis RM. Conservative management of childhood orbital lymphangioma. *Ophthalmology* 1989;96:484–489.
6. Wright JE, Sullivan TJ, Garner A, Wulc AE, Moseley IF. Orbital venous anomalies. *Ophthalmology* 1997;104:905–913.
7. Lieb WE, Merton DA, Shields JA, Cohen SM, Mitchell DG, Goldberg BB. Color Doppler imaging in the demonstration of an orbital varix. *Br J Ophthalmol* 1990;74:305–308.

Lymphangioma—Clinical and Pathologic Features

Patients with lymphangioma can experience intermittent episodes of abrupt proptosis usually due to spontaneous or traumatic hemorrhage in the tumor and sometimes secondary to proliferation of lymphoid tissue in the tumor at the time of systemic infection.

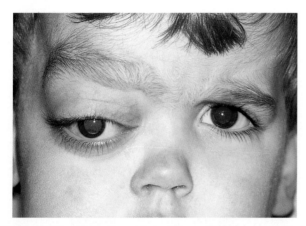

Figure 3-67. Proptosis and eyelid swelling in a 2-year-old boy with orbital lymphangioma.

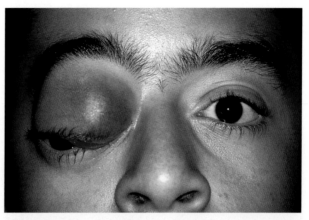

Figure 3-68. Mechanical blepharoptosis secondary to hemorrhage into the upper eyelid in a 14-year-old boy with lymphangioma. The tumor was occult until he developed sudden orbital hemorrhage following ocular trauma while playing basketball.

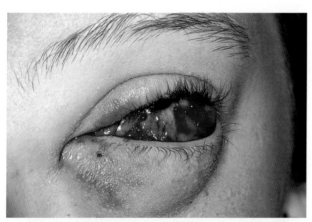

Figure 3-69. Conjunctival involvement by anterior extension of orbital lymphangioma allowing direct visualization of the lesion. Note the diffuse, cystic, hemorrhagic nature of the conjunctival component and the blue discoloration to the adjacent lower eyelid.

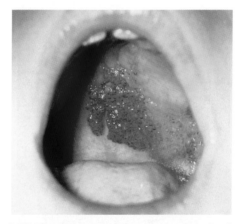

Figure 3-70. Involvement of the hard palate by lymphangioma in a patient with orbital lymphangioma. (Courtesy of Dr. Richard Margolies.)

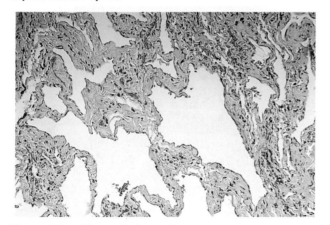

Figure 3-71. Histopathology of orbital lymphangioma showing bloodless, ectatic vascular channels with delicate connective tissue septa (hematoxylin–eosin, original magnification × 50).

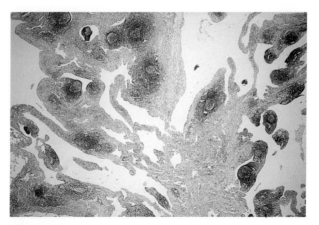

Figure 3-72. Histopathology of another case of orbital lymphangioma showing lymphoid tissue in the connective tissue septae. This lymphoid tissue, like the tonsils, is said to proliferate at the time of upper respiratory infections, worsening the proptosis.

Lymphangioma—Computed Tomography and Magnetic Resonance Imaging Features

Computed tomography and magnetic resonance imaging studies show very characteristic features in cases of orbital lymphangioma. There is an ill-defined multicystic mass with blood in many of the cysts.

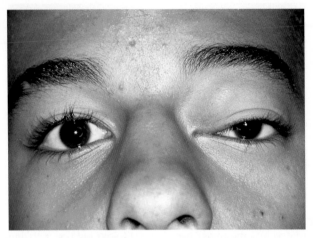

Figure 3-73. Blepharoptosis and fullness of the left upper eyelid in a 17-year-old boy.

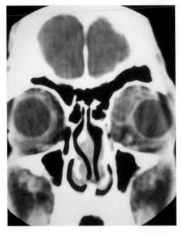

Figure 3-74. Coronal computed tomogram of the patient shown in Fig. 3-73 demonstrating the diffuse cystic mass superonasal to the globe.

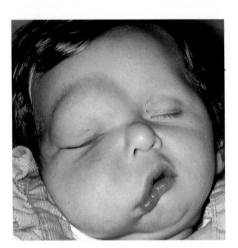

Figure 3-75. Massive orbital and subcutaneous lymphangioma around the right eye of a 3-month-old girl.

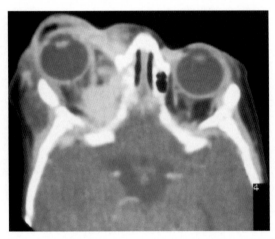

Figure 3-76. Axial computed tomogram of the child shown in Fig. 3-75 revealing diffuse orbital involvement by a multicystic mass.

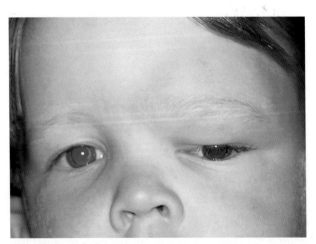

Figure 3-77. Orbital and periocular involvement of the left eye in a 3-year-old boy.

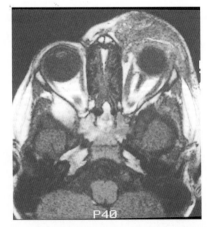

Figure 3-78. Axial magnetic resonance imaging of the child shown in Fig. 3-77 depicting a diffuse mass anterior and superior to the left eye. The lesion was presumed to be a lymphangioma, but a capillary hemangioma was considered a possibility. No biopsy was done.

Lymphangioma—Magnetic Resonance Imaging Features and Management by Aspiration

In some cases, a large hemorrhagic cyst can be identified and aspirated, which relieves the proptosis without the danger of extensive surgical intervention.

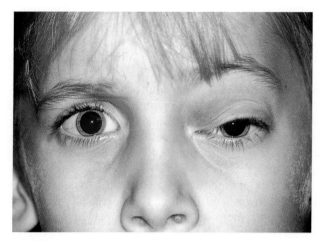

Figure 3-79. Blepharoptosis and fullness of the left upper eyelid and downward displacement of the left eye in an 8-year-old boy.

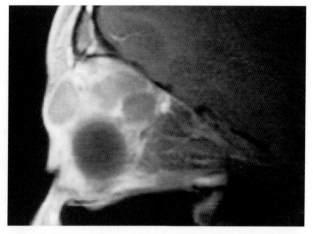

Figure 3-80. Sagittal magnetic resonance imaging in T1-weighted image of the child shown in Fig. 3-79 revealing an extensive multicystic mass involving most of the superior orbit.

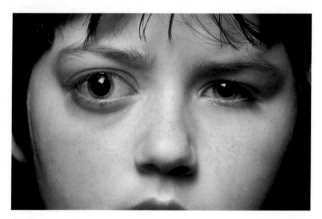

Figure 3-81. Proptosis of the right eye in an 11-year-old girl.

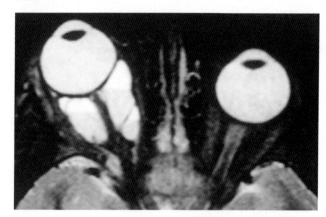

Figure 3-82. Axial magnetic resonance imaging in T2-weighted image of the child shown in Fig. 3-81 revealing large orbital cysts with a blood-fluid level.

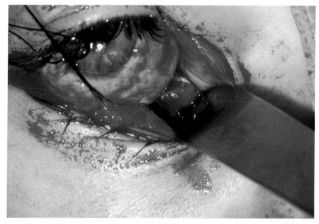

Figure 3-83. Identification of the blood-filled cyst shown in Fig. 3-82 following conjunctival forniceal incision and retraction of conjunctival and orbital tissue.

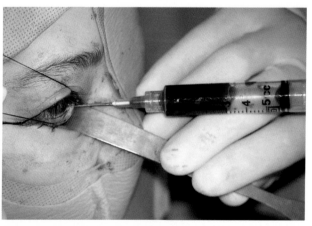

Figure 3-84. Aspiration of blood-filled cyst. This procedure brings about immediate reversal of the proptosis, and recurrence may take months or years.

VARIX

There is considerable overlap among orbital venous malformations, such as orbital varix, varicocele, and venous angioma, and they probably represent a spectrum of conditions. The differences among these conditions and the differences between a primary and secondary varix are discussed in the literature (1) and are beyond the scope of this atlas. Furthermore, there is controversy as to whether varix and lymphangioma represent the same entity (2,3). The authors believe that there are sufficient differences between them with regard to clinical and pathologic features to allow for separate classification (2). For purposes of this discussion, the term orbital varix is used to describe a mass produced by dilation of one or more orbital veins.

The classic varix usually becomes apparent in young adults and is characterized by positional proptosis, with the proptosis becoming worse with the head bent downward or during Valsalva maneuver. Computed tomography and magnetic resonance imaging demonstrate a round or irregular mass that may be relatively inapparent until Valsalva maneuver is performed during the scanning procedure (4). Color Doppler imaging also can be used to demonstrate an orbital varix (5).

Histopathologically, varix is seen as one or more dilated veins, frequently with thrombosis and hyalinization. Management is difficult and controversial. Minimally symptomatic lesions can be observed, and more symptomatic ones may require orbitotomy and surgical excision (1).

SELECTED REFERENCES

1. Shields JA. *Diagnosis and management of orbital tumors.* Philadelphia: WB Saunders, 1989:140–143.
2. Rootman J, Hay E, Graeb D, Miller R. Orbital-adnexal lymphangiomas. A spectrum of hemodynamically isolated vascular hamartomas. *Ophthalmology* 1986;93:1558–1570.
3. Wright JE, Sullivan TJ, Garner A, Wulc AE, Moseley IF. Orbital venous anomalies. *Ophthalmology* 1997;104:905–913.
4. Shields JA, Dolinskas C, Augsburger JJ, Shah HG, Shapiro ML. Demonstration of orbital varix with computed tomography and Valsalva maneuver. *Am J Ophthalmol* 1984;97:108–109.
5. Lieb WE, Merton DA, Shields JA, Cohen SM, Mitchell DG, Goldberg BB. Color Doppler imaging in the demonstration of an orbital varix. *Br J Ophthalmol* 1990;74:305–308.

Orbital Varix—Demonstration by Increasing Venous Pressure in the Head

In some instances, a subtle varix can show marked enlargement and increased proptosis during times of increased venous pressure in the head, induced by bending forward or by Valsalva maneuver. This can be demonstrated best by imaging studies with contrast enhancement.

From Shields JA, Dolinskas C, Augsburger JJ, Shah HG, Shapiro ML. Demonstration of orbital varix with computed tomography and Valsalva maneuver. *Am J Ophthalmol* 1984;97:108–109.

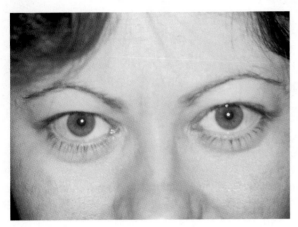

Figure 3-85. Minimal proptosis of the left eye in a 38-year-old woman who complains of a full feeling behind the left eye when she bends forward.

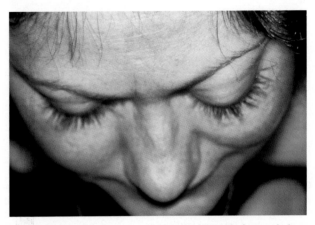

Figure 3-86. Appearance when patient bends forward showing more proptosis of the left eye.

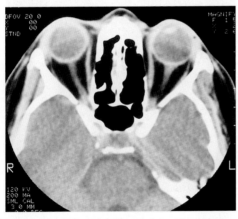

Figure 3-87. Axial computed tomogram of the same patient showing no apparent orbital mass.

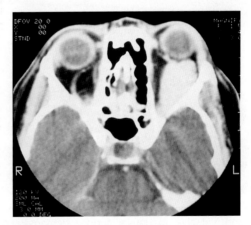

Figure 3-88. Axial computed tomogram of the same patient with contrast enhancement during Valsalva maneuver. Note that the enhancing orbital mass now is more prominent.

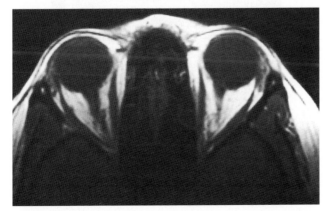

Figure 3-89. Axial magnetic resonance in T1-weighted image of the same patient showing no apparent mass.

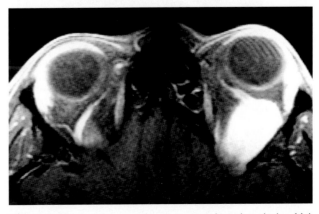

Figure 3-90. Axial magnetic resonance imaging during Valsalva maneuver demonstrated the mass.

Orbital Varix—Computed Tomography, Magnetic Resonance Imaging, and Color Doppler Imaging

In addition to computed tomography and magnetic resonance imaging, color Doppler imaging also can be employed to suggest the diagnosis of orbital varix.

Fig. 3-96 from Lieb WE, Merton DA, Shields JA, Cohen SM, Mitchell DG, Goldberg BB. Color Doppler imaging in the demonstration of an orbital varix. *Br J Ophthalmol* 1990;74:305–308.

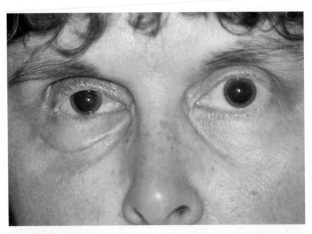

Figure 3-91. Slight enophthalmos of the right eye in 59-year-old woman who was referred after she had undergone three right orbitotomies to rule out orbital metastasis but no diagnosis had been established.

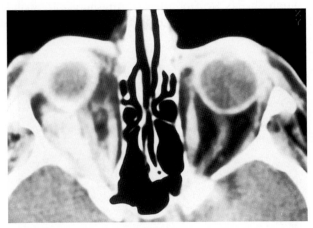

Figure 3-92. Axial computed tomogram with contrast agent and Valsalva maneuver demonstrating an enhancing mass near the floor of the orbit.

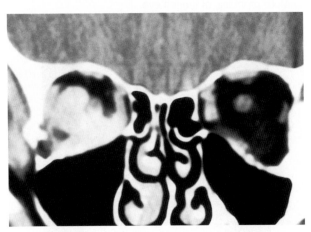

Figure 3-93. Coronal computed tomogram with contrast agent and Valsalva maneuver further demonstrating the mass.

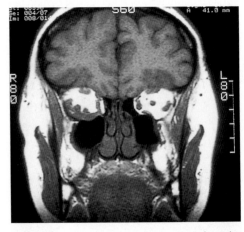

Figure 3-94. Coronal magnetic resonance imaging in T1-weighted image showing an irregular mass along the floor of the right orbit.

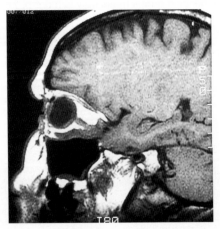

Figure 3-95. Sagittal magnetic resonance imaging in T1-weighted image further demonstrating the mass.

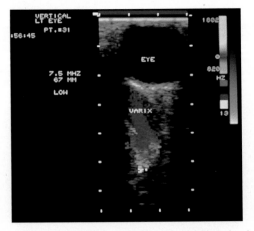

Figure 3-96. Color Doppler imaging of orbital varix showing the dilated retrobulbar vein as shown in blue.

Orbital Varix—Anteriorly Located Lesion

A varix located in the anterior aspects of the orbit can be clinically apparent through the eyelid or conjunctiva.

Fig. 3-99 through 3-102 from Shields JA, Eagle RC Jr, Shields CL, De Potter P, Shapiro RS. Orbital varix presenting as a subconjunctival mass. *Ophthal Plast Reconstr Surg* 1995;11:37–38.

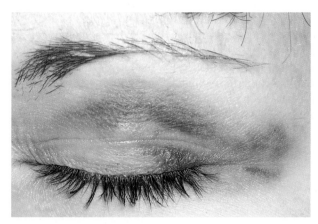

Figure 3-97. Subcutaneous ecchymosis around the left eye in a 36-year-old woman with bleeding from an orbital varix that had undergone thrombosis.

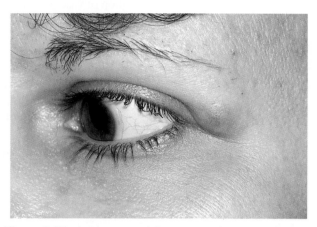

Figure 3-98. Appearance of the same patient 6 months later after the subcutaneous hemorrhage had resolved. Note that the thrombosed varix appears as a blue nodule beneath the skin near the lateral canthus.

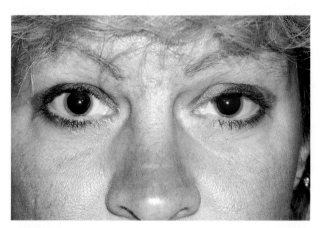

Figure 3-99. Slight blepharoptosis of the left eye in a 40-year-old woman.

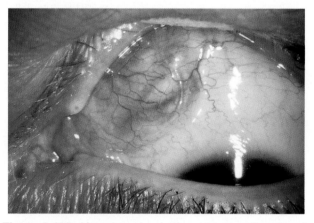

Figure 3-100. Vascular mass in the superonasal conjunctival fornix in the same patient shown in Fig. 3-99.

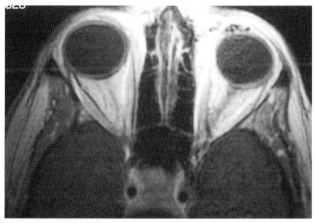

Figure 3-101. Axial magnetic resonance imaging of the patient shown in Fig. 3-99 demonstrating the irregular vascular mass in the anteromedial aspect of the orbit.

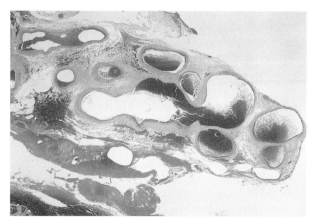

Figure 3-102. Histopathology of the same lesion shown in Fig. 3-101 demonstrated complex arrangement of dilated veins (hematoxylin–eosin, original magnification × 20).

INTRAVASCULAR PAPILLARY ENDOTHELIAL HYPERPLASIA AND GLOMUS TUMOR

Miscellaneous orbital vascular lesions to be covered here include intravascular papillary endothelial hyperplasia and glomus tumor. Intravascular papillary endothelial hyperplasia is a benign process composed of endothelial cells that undergo proliferation in a papillary configuration. It is possible that it represents an exuberant proliferation of vascular endothelium as a cellular response to the organization of a thrombus, possibly within an varix or arteriovenous communication. Clinically and radiographically, it appears as a circumscribed mass similar to cavernous hemangioma and hemangiopericytoma. The management is surgical excision (1–4).

Glomus cell tumor (glomangioma) is a vascular lesion that arises from the glomus body, a specialized structure that has a thermoregulatory function. It can occasionally occur in the eyelid (5,6). It also has been recognized in the orbit, where it simulates other circumscribed orbital tumors (7). The best management is surgical excision.

SELECTED REFERENCES

1. Shields JA. *Diagnosis and management of orbital tumors.* Philadelphia: WB Saunders, 1989:143–145.
2. Font RL, Wheeler TM, Boniuk M. Intravascular papillary endothelial hyperplasia of the orbit and ocular adnexa. A report of five cases. *Arch Ophthalmol* 1983;101:1731–1736.
3. Weber FL, Babel J. Intravascular papillary endothelial hyperplasia of the orbit. *Br J Ophthalmol* 1981;65: 18–22.
4. Shields JA, Shields CL, Diniz W, Eagle RC Jr. Multiple bilateral orbital vascular tumors as a component of intravascular papillary endothelial hyperplasia (*submitted*).
5. Charles NC. Multiple glomus tumors of the face and eyelid. *Arch Ophthalmol* 1976;94:1283–1285.
6. Saxe SJ, Grossniklaus HE, Wojno TH, Hertzler GL, Boniuk M, Font RL. Glomus cell tumor of the eyelid. *Ophthalmology* 1993;100:139–143.
7. Neufeld M, Pe'er J, Rosenman E, Lazar M. Intraorbital glomus cell tumor. *Am J Ophthalmol* 1994;117: 539–540.

Intravascular Papillary Endothelial Hyperplasia and Glomus Tumor

Figs. 3-103 through 3-105 from Shields JA, Shields CL, Diniz W, Eagle RC Jr. Multiple bilateral orbital vascular tumors as a component of intravascular papillary endothelial hyperplasia (*submitted*).

Figs. 3-106 through 3-108 courtesy of Dr. Jacob Pe'er. From Neufeld M, Pe'er J, Rosenman E, Lazar M. Intraorbital glomus cell tumor. *Am J Ophthalmol* 1994;117: 539–540.

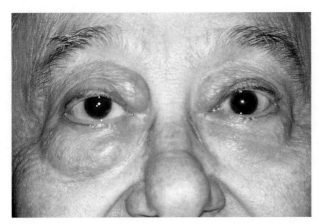

Figure 3-103. Intravascular papillary endothelial hyperplasia causing proptosis and eyelid edema of the right eye in an otherwise healthy 80-year-old woman.

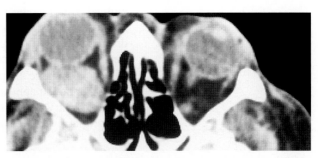

Figure 3-104. Axial computed tomogram of the patient shown in Fig. 3-103 demonstrating a circumscribed retrobulbar tumor resembling a cavernous hemangioma. Addtional sections showed similar but smaller masses at the right orbital apex in the soft tissues of the left orbit.

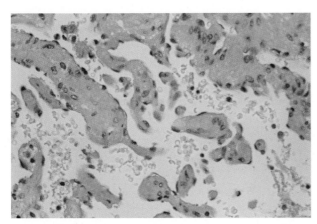

Figure 3-105. Histopathology of the lesion shown in Fig. 3-104 depicting projections of proliferating endothelial cells into the lumen of a vascular channel (hematoxylin–eosin, original magnification × 100).

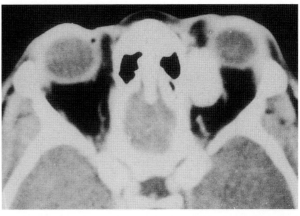

Figure 3-106. Axial computed tomogram of an intraorbital glomus cell tumor in a 35-year-old woman showing a circumscribed mass in the superonasal aspect of the left orbit.

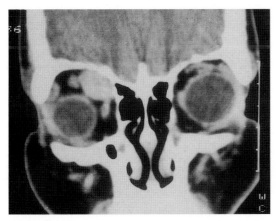

Figure 3-107. Coronal computed tomogram of the lesion shown in Fig. 3-106.

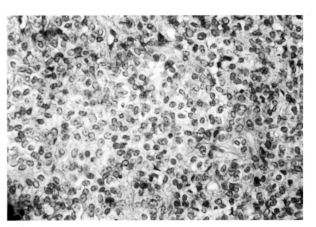

Figure 3-108. Histopathology of the lesion shown in Fig. 3-106 revealing sheets of polyhedral cells. Immunohistochemical studies supported the diagnosis of glomus tumor (hematoxylin–eosin, original magnification × 125).

ANGIOSARCOMA

Angiosarcoma (malignant hemangioendothelioma) is a malignant tumor that probably arises from endothelial cells of blood vessels. Angiosarcoma that arises in the orbit has the capacity to invade locally but it rarely metastasizes (1–5). It has a tendency to occur in young adults. It can be localized or diffuse, and it has no distinct clinical or radiologic features that serve to differentiate it from other orbital tumors. Angiosarcoma near the orbital apex has been known to produce a Tolosa–Hunt syndrome, with painful ophthalmoplegia (3). It can extend from the orbit into the conjunctiva and resemble Kaposi's sarcoma of the conjunctiva (4). Histopathologically, it can occur as large anaplastic cells that proliferate into the vascular lumen, giving it a pseudoglandular appearance, or it can occur as an epithelioid cell variant (3). Immunohistochemistry or electron microscopy may be required to demonstrate the endothelial cell origin in some cases (3,4).

SELECTED REFERENCES

1. Shields JA. *Diagnosis and management of orbital tumors.* Philadelphia: WB Saunders, 1989:138–140.
2. Carelli PV, Cangelosi JP. Angiosarcoma of the orbit. *Am J Ophthalmol* 1948;31:453–456.
3. Messmer EP, Font RL, McCrary JA, et al. Epithelioid angiosarcoma of the orbit presenting as Tolosa–Hunt Syndrome. *Ophthalmology* 1983;90:1414–1421.
4. Hufnagel T, Ma L, Kuo T. Orbital angiosarcoma with subconjunctival presentation. *Ophthalmology* 1987;94: 72–77.
5. Gunduz K, Shields JA, Shields CL, Eagle RC Jr, Nathan F. Cutaneous angiosarcoma with eyelid involvement. *Am J Ophthalmol* 1998;125:870–871.

Angiosarcoma

Figs. 3-111 through 3-114 courtesy of Dr. Ramon Font. From Messmer EP, Font RL, McCrary JA, et al. Epithelioid angiosarcoma of the orbit presenting as Tolosa–Hunt Syndrome. *Ophthalmology* 1983;90:1414–1421.

AUTHOR'S NOTE: Several years later, immunohistochemical studies suggested that the tumor reported by Messmer et al. possibly was an example of invasive squamous cell carcinoma (personal communication, Dr. Ramon Font, 1998).

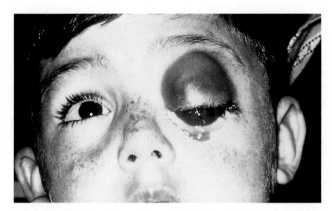

Figure 3-109. Angiosarcoma of the left orbit with secondary eyelid and conjunctival involvement in a young boy. (Courtesy of Dr. Frederick Blodi.)

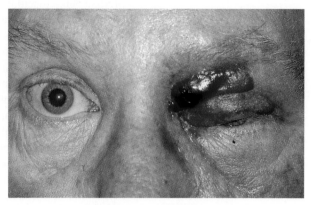

Figure 3-110. Angiosarcoma of the left orbit with secondary extension into the eyelid in a 70-year-old man.

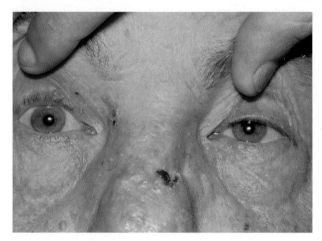

Figure 3-111. Proptosis of the left eye secondary to an epithelioid angiosarcoma of the orbit that produced a Tolosa–Hunt syndrome.

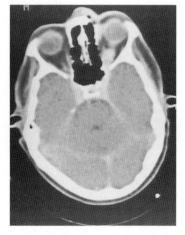

Figure 3-112. Axial computed tomogram of the patient shown in Fig. 3-111 demonstrating an irregular mass near the orbital apex.

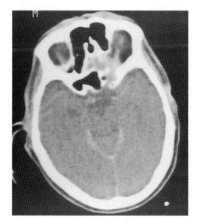

Figure 3-113. Axial computed tomogram of a section more inferior of the lesion shown in Fig. 3-112 demonstrating extensive bone destruction near the orbital apex.

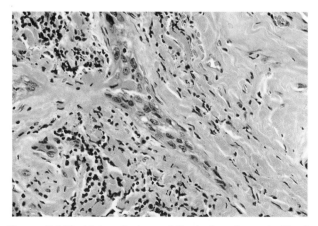

Figure 3-114. Histopathology of the lesion shown in Fig. 3-112 demonstrating malignant endothelial cells with fibrous tissue stroma (hematoxylin–eosin, original magnification × 200).

ORGANIZING HEMATOMA

Orbital hematoma is not a vascular tumor but rather a localized accumulation of blood that results from bleeding from an abnormal or damaged blood vessel. In a prior textbook, we included it under the name of hematocele in the chapter on orbital cysts (1). However, orbital hematoma is not a true cyst because it lacks an epithelial lining. Henderson (2) provides a convincing argument for using the term organizing hematoma, phraseology that we have adopted here. Although there can be a number of predisposing vascular lesions, particularly lymphangioma and varix, the majority of orbital hematomas are a result of trauma. The patient often presents with either an abrupt or gradual onset and progression of unilateral proptosis and downward displacement of the globe. Some patients recall a history or prior trauma with eyelid ecchymosis, which may have occurred months or years earlier. The reason for this delay in onset of symptoms is unclear.

In the most common type of organizing traumatic hematoma, computed tomography and magnetic resonance imaging typically show a circumscribed mass in the superior aspect of the orbit with contents compatible with organizing blood. It usually is located between the periorbitum and superior orbital bone, accounting for its well-defined margin. An organizing hematoma in the superior orbit can sometimes erode through the bone and encroach on the brain. Histopathologically, organizing hematoma is characterized by altered blood in various stages of degeneration and organization, with accumulation of cholesterol and a bile pigment called hematoidin. Although some hematomas resolve on their own, many of them that become symptomatic show progressive enlargement, perhaps due to an osmotic gradient created by the blood products, which allows more absorption of fluid and increase in size. The treatment is surgical excision by evacuating the blood and its fibrous tissue capsule. When the tumor extends into the cranial cavity, the procedure often is undertaken in conjunction with a neurosurgeon.

SELECTED REFERENCES

1. Shields JA. *Diagnosis and management of orbital tumors.* Philadelphia: WB Saunders, 1989:115–117.
2. Henderson JW. *Orbital tumors*, 3rd ed. New York: Raven Press, 1994:73–78.

Organizing Hematoma

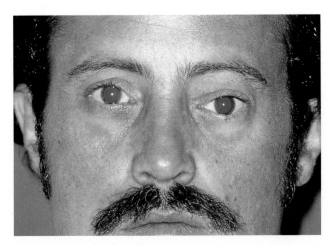

Figure 3-115. Proptosis and downward displacement of the left eye in a 31-year-old man.

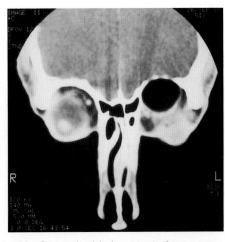

Figure 3-116. Coronal orbital computed tomogram showing homogeneous circumscribed mass, compatible with blood, in the superior orbit.

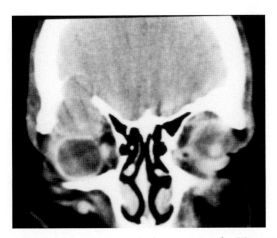

Figure 3-117. Coronal computed tomogram of a 32-year-old man with a history of prior ocular trauma. Note the superior orbital mass that displaces the globe downward and extends through the orbital roof into the cranial cavity. This was found histopathologically to be an organizing hematoma.

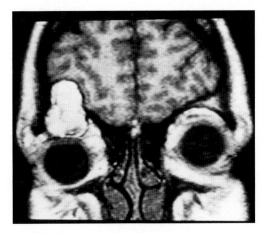

Figure 3-118. Coronal magnetic resonance imaging of the same patient shown in Fig. 3-117 delineating the organizing hematoma.

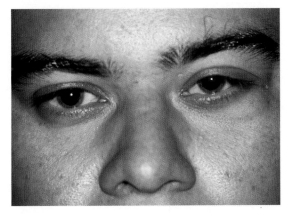

Figure 3-119. Proptosis and slight upward displacement of the right eye in a 26-year-old man.

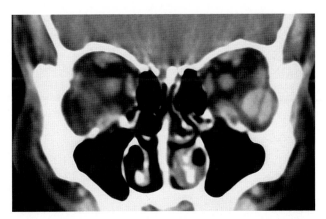

Figure 3-120. Coronal computed tomogram of the patient shown in Fig. 3-119 revealing a circumscribed inferotemporal orbital mass. It proved pathologically to be an organizing hematoma with a dense fibrous pseudocapsule.

CHAPTER 4

Peripheral Nerve Tumors

NEURILEMOMA (SCHWANNOMA)

Some tumors that arise from the orbital peripheral nerves include neurilemoma, neurofibroma, alveolar soft-part sarcoma, granular cell tumor, malignant peripheral nerve-sheath tumor, and amputation neuroma.

Neurilemoma (schwannoma) is a benign tumor that arises from Schwann cells that ensheath peripheral nerves. Although it accounted for only 1% of all orbital biopsies in the authors' series (1,2), a number of such cases subsequently have been identified, and it may be more common than reflected in that series. Orbital neurilemoma usually occurs in young to middle-aged adults and produces noninflammatory proptosis and displacement of the globe with signs and symptoms similar to those described for orbital cavernous hemangioma. Even though it is a tumor of peripheral nerve-sheath origin, it rarely produces pain. Imaging studies disclose a solid mass, usually outside the muscle cone along the course of the supraorbital or supratrochlear nerve and occasionally along the infraorbital nerve. The tumor frequently is ovoid or elongated, reflecting its course along the nerve (1–4).

Histopathologically, neurilemoma can show several variations, but it usually is composed of a benign proliferation of Schwann cells. It may appear as ribbons or fascicles of spindle cells (Antoni A pattern) or as more ovoid clear cells (Antoni B pattern). Although there are no good immunohistochemical stains that are specific for Schwann cells, immunohistochemistry can be used to exclude the diagnosis of other spindle cell tumors, such as melanoma, leiomyoma, and rhabdomyosarcoma, thus lending support to the diagnosis of neurilemoma. Electron microscopy can be used to demonstrate the cytoplasmic wide-spacing collagen that characterizes Schwann cells (Luse bodies). The management of orbital neurilemoma is surgical excision. An incisional biopsy generally should not be done for this circumscribed orbital tumor. If the tumor is not completely excised at a fairly early stage, it can show progressive growth and attain a large size, and thus be more difficult to excise.

SELECTED REFERENCES

1. Shields JA, Bakewell B, Augsburger DG, Flanagan JC. Classification and incidence of space-occupying lesions of the orbit. A survey of 645 biopsies. *Arch Ophthalmol* 1984;102:1606–1611.
2. Shields JA. *Diagnosis and management of orbital tumors.* Philadelphia: WB Saunders, 1989:152–157.
3. Rootman J, Goldberg C, Robertson W. Primary orbital schwannomas. *Br J Ophthalmol* 1982;66:194–204.
4. Shields JA, Kapustiak J, Arbizo V, Augsburger JJ, Schnitzer RE. Orbital neurilemoma with extension through the superior orbital fissure. *Arch Ophthalmol* 1986;104:871–873.

Neurilemoma

Orbital neurilemoma most typically occurs in the superior extraconal portion of the orbit and apparently arises from the sheath of the supraorbital nerve. It is best approached by a superolateral orbitotomy. Most can be removed successfully by a soft-tissue approach. An osteotomy only occasionally is necessary. A clinicopathologic correlation is presented.

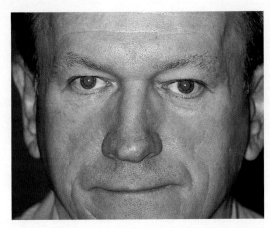

Figure 4-1. Proptosis and downward displacement of the left eye in a 57-year-old man.

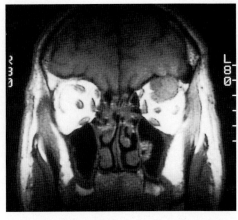

Figure 4-2. Coronal magnetic resonance imaging in T1-weighted image showing circumscribed superior orbital mass.

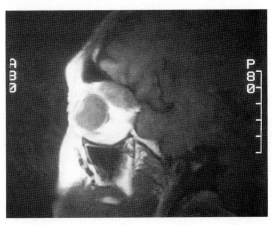

Figure 4-3. Sagittal magnetic resonance imaging in T1-weighted image showing ovoid shape of the superior orbital mass.

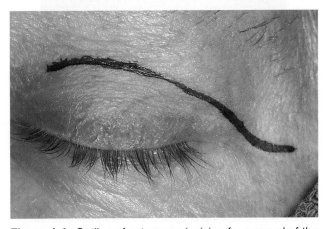

Figure 4-4. Outline of cutaneous incision for removal of the mass. The lesion was removed without complications.

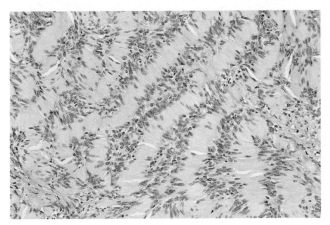

Figure 4-5. Histopathology showing an area of Antoni A pattern with fascicles of nuclei with a ribbon arrangement (hematoxylin–eosin, original magnification × 150).

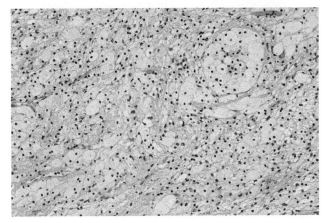

Figure 4-6. Histopathology of another area of the same tumor showing Antoni B pattern (hematoxylin–eosin, original magnification × 150).

Orbital neurilemoma is a benign, slowly growing tumor that can cause compression of the optic nerve and visual impairment. Once the tumor is removed, optic disc swelling can resolve and visual acuity can return to normal. An example is illustrated.

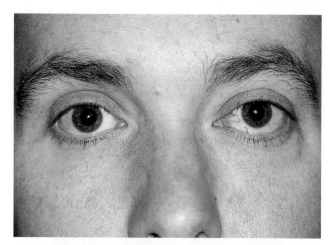

Figure 4-7. Proptosis of the left eye in a 29-year-old man.

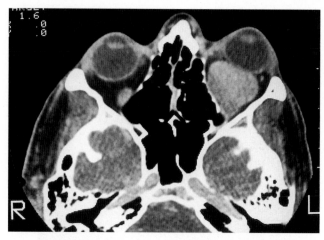

Figure 4-8. Axial computed tomography showing a large superior orbital mass. Other sections showed compression of the optic nerve.

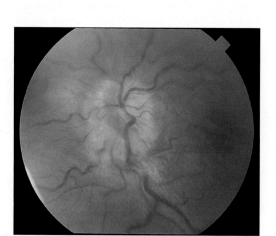

Figure 4-9. Fundus photograph showing edema of the left optic nerve, tortuous retinal blood vessels, and choroidal folds. Visual acuity was 6/60.

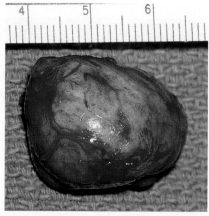

Figure 4-10. Gross appearance of the circumscribed tumor immediately after removal through a superolateral orbitotomy.

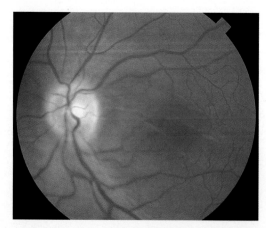

Figure 4-11. Fundus photograph taken 6 months later showing disappearance of the optic disc edema and reversal of the retinal vascular tortuosity. The visual acuity had returned to 6/6. The choroidal folds persisted.

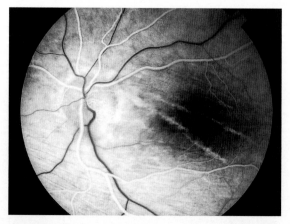

Figure 4-12. Fluorescein angiogram in the arterial phase, 6 months after surgery, showing transmission hyperfluorescence through the persistent choroidal folds.

Because orbital neurilemoma is a well-circumscribed, encapsulated tumor, it sometimes can be removed intact via lateral orbitotomy in spite of a large size and posterior location. A clinicopathologic correlation of a large neurilemoma in a 33-year-old man who declined a recommended neurosurgical approach and sought another opinion to see if it could be removed without a craniotomy is illustrated. The neurilemoma was removed intact via a superolateral orbitotomy in spite of the fact that it protruded posteriorly through the superior orbital fissure.

From Shields JA, Kapustiak J, Arbizo V, Augsburger JJ, Schnitzer RE. Orbital neurilemoma with extension through the superior orbital fissure. *Arch Ophthalmol* 1986;104:871–873.

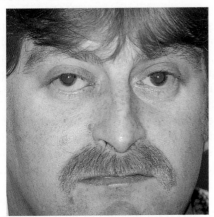

Figure 4-13. Clinical appearance showing proptosis of the right eye.

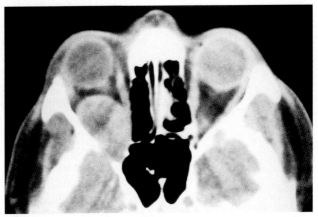

Figure 4-14. Axial computed tomography showing large circumscribed mass occupying most of posterior orbit and extending through the superior orbital fissure into the brain.

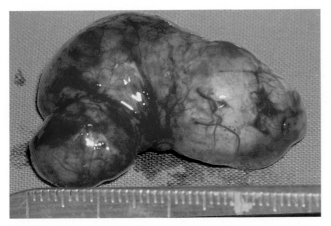

Figure 4-15. Appearance of the mass immediately after removal by orbitotomy. The nodular protrusion corresponded to where the tumor protruded posteriorly through the superior orbital fissure.

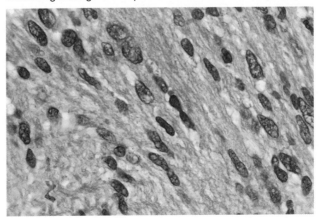

Figure 4-16. Histopathology of an area of tumor showing neurilemoma with Antoni A pattern (hematoxylin–eosin, original magnification × 200).

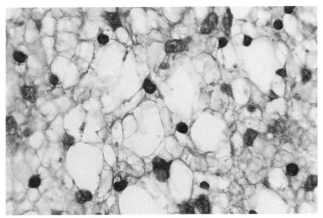

Figure 4-17. Histopathology of another area of the tumor showing Antoni B pattern (hematoxylin–eosin, original magnification × 200).

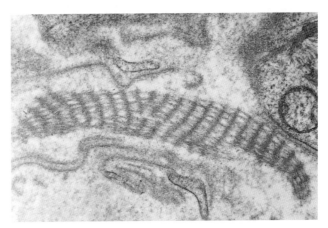

Figure 4-18. Electron photomicrograph of tumor showing wide-spacing collagen in the cytoplasm (Luse body).

NEUROFIBROMA

Neurofibroma is a benign, peripheral nerve tumor that is composed of a combined proliferation of Schwann cells, endoneural fibroblasts, and axons. It accounted for about 1% of biopsied orbital tumors in the authors' series (1,2). Neurofibroma can be divided into localized, diffuse, and plexiform types. The localized type has a low, but definite, association with neurofibromatosis, and the latter almost always is seen in association with neurofibromatosis. Plexiform neurofibroma is generally a diffuse tumor, and the localized neurofibroma usually is well circumscribed (3–7). The diffuse type can occur as multiple tumors, in which case it may represent a manifestation of neurofibromatosis type 2. Orbital neurofibroma associated with neurofibromatosis can be very extensive, with massive involvement of the orbit, eyelids, conjunctiva, uveal tract, and surrounding periocular tissues. In addition, patients with neurofibromatosis can have congenital defects in the sphenoid bone that can produce a characteristic pulsating proptosis similar to that seen with encephalocele.

Histopathologically, diffuse and plexiform neurofibromas are composed of intertwining bundles of enlarged nerves with proliferation of Schwann cells and endoneural fibroblasts in a mucoid matrix. A distinct perineural sheath defines the individual tumor cores. The localized neurofibroma lacks a perineural sheath and is encapsulated. As for neurilemoma, the management of localized neurofibroma is complete surgical resection. The diffuse unresectable plexiform type should be managed more conservatively. However, surgical intervention is often necessary because of bothersome symptoms, threatened vision, or an unacceptable cosmetic appearance. In such instances, debulking surgery often is done, because complete surgical removal may not be possible.

SELECTED REFERENCES

1. Shields JA, Bakewell B, Augsburger DG, Flanagan CJ. Classification and incidence of space-occupying lesions of the orbit. A survey of 645 biopsies. *Arch Ophthalmol* 1984;102:1606–1611.
2. Shields JA. *Diagnosis and management of orbital tumors.* Philadelphia: WB Saunders Co, 1989:149–152.
3. Brownstein S, Little JM. Ocular neurofibromatosis. *Ophthalmology* 1983;91:1595–1599.
4. Krohel GB, Rosenberg PN, Wright JE, et al. Localized orbital neurofibromas. *Am J Ophthalmol* 1985;100: 458–464.
5. Kobrin JL, Blodi FC, Weingeist TA, et al. Ocular and orbital manifestations of neurofibromatosis. *Surv Ophthalmol* 1979;24:45–51.
6. Shields JA, Shields CL, Lieb WE, Eagle RC Jr. Multiple orbital neurofibromas unassociated with von Recklinghausen's disease. *Arch Ophthalmol* 1990;108:80–83.
7. De Potter P, Shields CL, Shields JA, Rao VM, Eagle RC Jr, Trachtenberg WM. The CT and MRI features of an unusual case of isolated orbital neurofibroma. *J Ophthal Reconstr Plast Surg* 1992;8:221–227.

Orbital Involvement with Neurofibromatosis

Patients with neurofibromatosis can develop a plexiform or a diffuse neurofibroma of the orbit, as well as juvenile pilocytic astrocytoma of the optic nerve, to be discussed in Chapter 5. Another orbital manifestation is pulsating proptosis secondary to absence of the greater wing of the sphenoid bone.

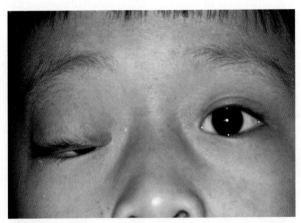

Figure 4-19. Blepharoptosis and proptosis of the right eye in a 6-year-old boy with plexiform neurofibroma of the orbit.

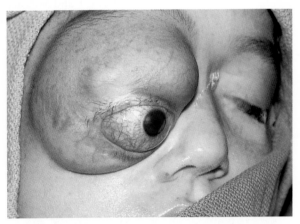

Figure 4-20. More extensive orbital neurofibroma in an 8-year-old girl. (Courtesy of Dr. Bruce Johnson.)

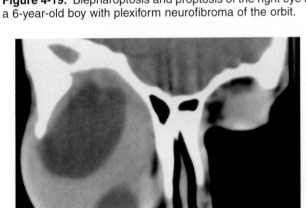

Figure 4-21. Coronal computed tomography of the patient shown in Fig. 4-20 demonstrating the large orbital mass with clear areas that probably represent mucinous degeneration in the tumor. (Courtesy of Dr. Bruce Johnson.)

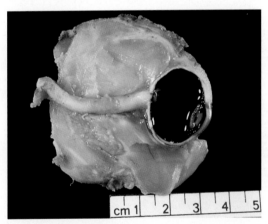

Figure 4-22. Gross appearance of the lesion shown in Fig. 4-20 following orbital exenteration. Note the advanced diffuse orbital tumor and the long section of grossly normal optic nerve. (Courtesy of Dr. Bruce Johnson.)

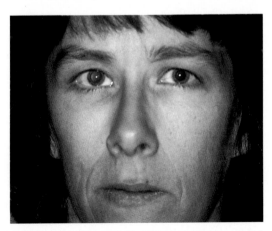

Figure 4-23. Appearance of a 35-year-old woman with neurofibromatosis. She had pulsations of the right eye but minimal proptosis.

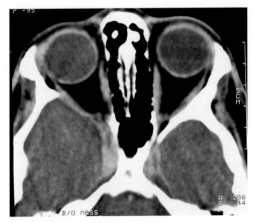

Figure 4-24. Axial computed tomography of the patient shown in Fig. 4-23. Note the absence of the sphenoid bone, which allows brain pulsations to be transmitted to the orbit.

Solitary Orbital Neurofibroma

Solitary orbital neurofibroma can occur in the orbit of adults, often unassociated with neurofibromatosis. A clinicopathologic correlation with computed tomography and magnetic resonance imaging in a 35-year-old woman is illustrated.

From De Potter P, Shields CL, Shields JA, Rao VM, Eagle RC Jr, Trachtenberg WM. The CT and MRI features of an unusual case of isolated orbital neurofibroma. *J Ophthal Reconstr Plast Surg* 1992;8:221–227.

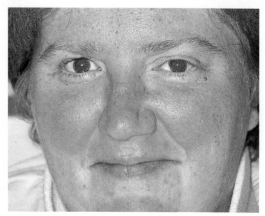

Figure 4-25. Facial appearance showing proptosis of the left eye.

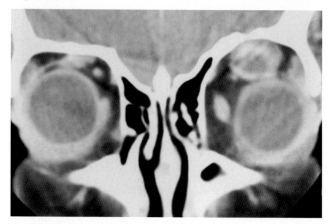

Figure 4-26. Coronal computed tomography showing superior orbital mass with cyst-like central portion.

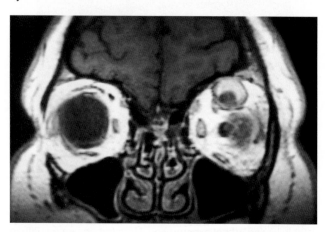

Figure 4-27. Coronal magnetic resonance imaging in T1-weighted image showing the superior orbital mass with low-signal component.

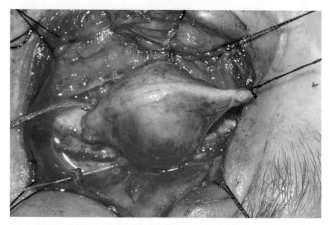

Figure 4-28. Appearance of the mass at the time of surgical exposure. Note the visible nerve coursing along the margin of the mass.

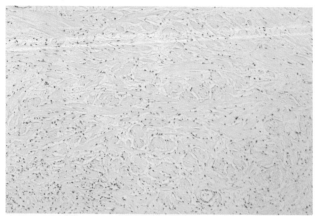

Figure 4-29. Histopathology of the tumor showing large eosinophilic nerve bundles (hematoxylin–eosin, original magnification × 75).

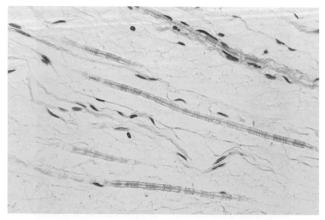

Figure 4-30. Histopathology showing area of extensive mucinous degeneration, corresponding to the low-signal component seen on magnetic resonance imaging and computed tomography (hematoxylin–eosin, original magnification × 75).

Multiple Circumscribed Orbital Neurofibromas

Multiple separate neurofibromas can develop in one orbit, apparently unassociated with neurofibromatosis. In the 58-year-old man illustrated here, there was no clinical evidence of neurofibromatosis except for three separate neurofibromas in the right orbit. It is possible that it could represent a *forme fruste* of von Recklinghausen's neurofibromatosis. The patient's chronic pain completely resolved after surgical removal of the tumors.

From Shields JA, Shields CL, Lieb WE, Eagle RC Jr. Multiple orbital neurofibromas unassociated with von Recklinghausen's disease. *Arch Ophthalmol* 1990;108:80–83.

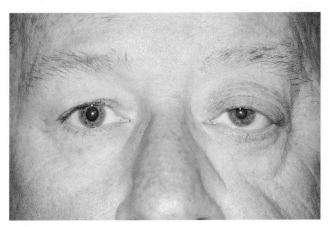

Figure 4-31. Proptosis of the right eye, which had been slowly progressive and painful for several years.

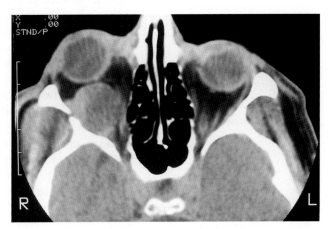

Figure 4-32. Axial computed tomography showing retrobulbar mass and a separate mass in the temporal fossa.

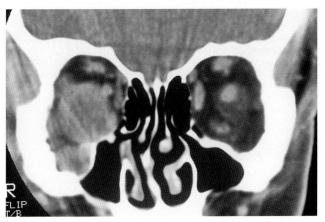

Figure 4-33. Coronal computed tomography showing the retrobulbar mass and a third mass in the inferior aspect of the orbit with displacement of the bony floor of the orbit.

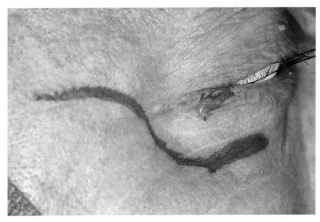

Figure 4-34. Skin incision line for inferolateral orbitotomy. Three separate masses were removed intact via this approach.

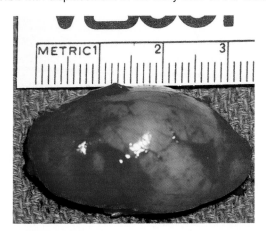

Figure 4-35. Appearance of the retrobulbar mass immediately after surgical removal of all three tumors. Note that the lesion is greater than 30 mm in length.

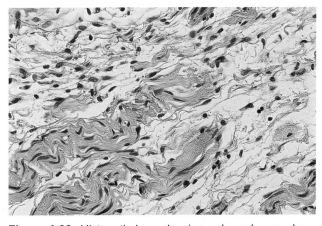

Figure 4-36. Histopathology showing enlarged nerve bundles in a mucoid stroma (hematoxylin–eosin, original magnification × 150).

ALVEOLAR SOFT-PART SARCOMA

Alveolar soft-part sarcoma is a soft-tissue neoplasm of disputed origin that can occur in the orbit, usually in young children and less often in young adults (1–5). The affected patient usually presents with rather rapid onset and progression of proptosis, a course similar to the more common orbital rhabdomyosarcoma (see Chapter 6). In the early stages, the tumor is small and circumscribed. If not treated early and effectively, it can become alarmingly aggressive and can fill the orbit and destroy the globe. In the early stages, imaging studies show a circumscribed mass; in the later stages, it is a diffuse, poorly defined mass. Histopathology shows large, round to polyhedral cells that assume a pseudoalveolar pattern with the alveolar spaces separated by delicate fibrovascular trabeculae. The loosely cohesive cells sometimes float freely in the alveolar spaces, resembling the alveolar variant of rhabdomyosarcoma. A characteristic feature is the presence of typical periodic acid–Schiff-positive diastase-resistant intracytoplasmic crystalline structures that can be demonstrated with electron microscopy. The pathogenesis is still a matter of debate. A leading possibility is that it represents a tumor of neural origin, perhaps a malignant variant of a paraganglioma (chemodectoma) or granular cell tumor (1,2).

The management is wide surgical excision followed by irradiation and chemotherapy, similar to the treatment of rhabdomyosarcoma. Metastatis can occur, usually to the lungs. In a series of 17 cases, two patients died from metastatic disease (1).

SELECTED REFERENCES

1. Font RL, Jurco S, Zimmerman LE. Alveolar soft-part sarcoma of the orbit: a clinicopathologic analysis of seventeen cases and a review of the literature. *Hum Pathol* 1982;13:569–579.
2. Shields JA. *Diagnosis and management of orbital tumors.* Philadelphia: WB Saunders, 1989:161–163.
3. Grant GD, Shields JA, Flanagan JC, Horowitz P. The ultrasonographic and radiologic features of a histologically proven case of alveolar soft-part sarcoma of the orbit. *Am J Ophthalmol* 1979;87:773–777.
4. Bunt AH, Bensinger RE. Alveolar soft-part sarcoma of the orbit. *Ophthalmology* 1981;888:1339–1346.
5. Jordan DR, MacDonald H, Noel L, Carpenter B, Brownstein S, Munro S. Alveolar soft-part sarcoma of the orbit. *Ophthalmic Surg* 1995;26;269–270.

Alveolar Soft-part Sarcoma

Figs. 4-37 through 4-39 from Grant GD, Shields JA, Flanagan JC, Horowitz P. The ultrasonographic and radiologic features of a histologically proven case of alveolar soft-part sarcoma of the orbit. *Am J Ophthalmol* 1979;87:773–777.

Figs. 4-40 through 4-42 courtesy of Dr. Seymour Brownstein. From Jordan DR, MacDonald H, Noel L, Carpenter B, Brownstein S, Munro S. Alveolar soft-part sarcoma of the orbit. *Ophthalmic Surg* 1995;26;269–270.

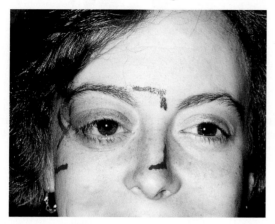

Figure 4-37. Proptosis of the right eye in an 18-year-old woman. A biopsy has been done and the face has been marked in preparation for radiotherapy.

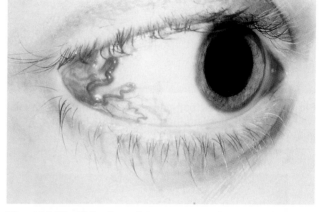

Figure 4-38. Side view of the right eye of the patient shown in Fig. 4-37 disclosing large, dilated, episcleral blood vessels temporally.

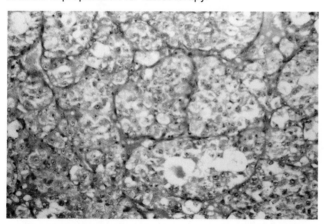

Figure 4-39. Histopathology of the tumor from the patient shown in Fig. 4-37 demonstrating the alveolar arrangement of the cells (hematoxylin–eosin, original magnification × 100).

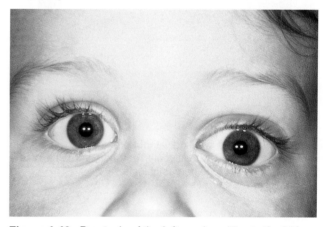

Figure 4-40. Proptosis of the left eye in a 19-month-old boy.

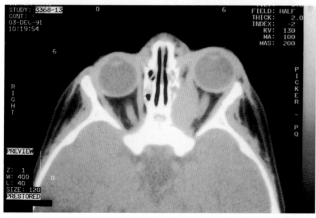

Figure 4-41. Axial computed tomography of the patient shown in Fig. 4-40 demonstrating a solid mass along the medial wall of the left orbit.

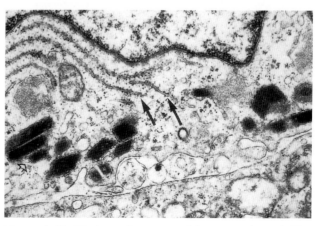

Figure 4-42. Electron microscopy of the tumor shown in Fig. 4-41 showing the characteristic crystalline inclusions in the cytoplasm *(arrows)* (original magnification × 10,000).

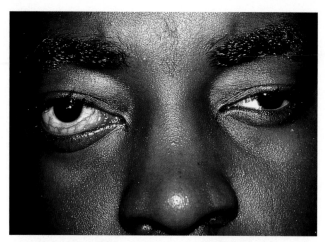

Figure 4-43. Alveolar soft-part sarcoma along the medial wall of the orbit affecting the medial rectus muscle in a 19-year-old man. (Courtesy of Dr. Victor Curtin.)

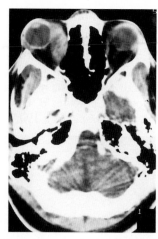

Figure 4-44. Axial computed tomography of the patient shown in Fig. 4-43 disclosing the medial right orbital mass. (Courtesy of Dr. Victor Curtin.)

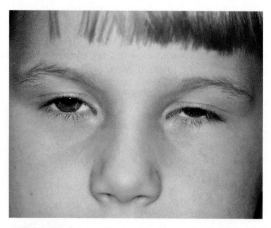

Figure 4-45. Eyelid swelling without proptosis of the left eye in a 6-year-old boy with alveolar soft-part sarcoma of the orbit. (Courtesy of Dr. Thomas Naugle.)

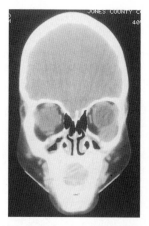

Figure 4-46. Axial computed tomography of the patient shown in Fig. 4-45 revealing an inferotemporal orbital mass on the left side. The mass was excised and found to be an alveolar soft-part sarcoma. (Courtesy of Dr. Thomas Naugle.)

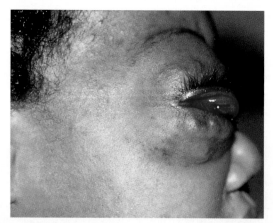

Figure 4-47. Proptosis and chemosis of the right eye in a 2-year-old boy with alveolar soft-part sarcoma of the orbit (Courtesy of Dr. Lorenz E. Zimmerman.).

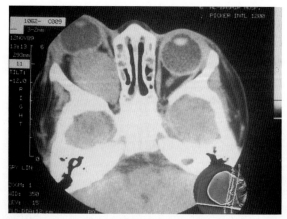

Figure 4-48. Axial computed tomography of the right orbit showing a large circumscribed orbital mass. The tumor was resected but it recurred, requiring orbital exenteration. (Courtesy of Dr. Lorenz E. Zimmerman.)

Aggressive Alveolar Soft-part Sarcoma

In some instances, alveolar soft-part sarcoma can be remarkably aggressive and attain a large size in spite of treatment efforts. This is shown in the clinicopathologic correlation illustrated here.

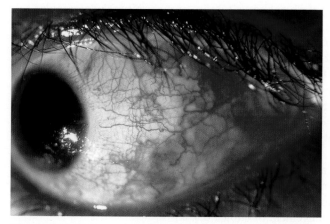

Figure 4-49. Dilated epibulbar blood vessels in the left eye of a 5-year-old child. (Courtesy of Dr. John D. Wright.)

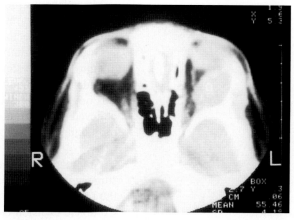

Figure 4-50. Axial computed tomography showing ovoid mass along the lateral wall of the orbit. The child was treated elsewhere with corticosteroids and diagnosed with orbital inflammatory pseudotumor, but the lesion continued to progress. Biopsy revealed alveolar soft-part sarcoma. (Courtesy of Dr. John D. Wright.)

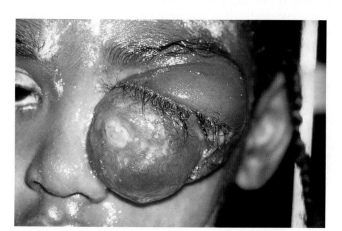

Figure 4-51. Appearance of the patient 3 months later showing marked progression of the lesion. (Courtesy of Dr. John D. Wright.)

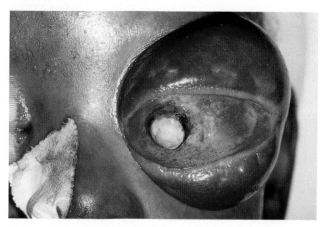

Figure 4-52. Appearance of the patient shown in Fig. 4-51, 3 months later, showing no improvement in spite of chemotherapy. Orbital exenteration was performed. (Courtesy of Dr. John D. Wright.)

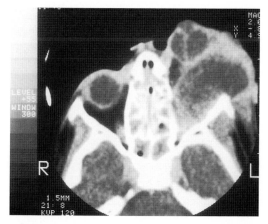

Figure 4-53. Axial computed tomography taken at time of the photograph shown in Fig. 4-52 disclosing a massive orbital tumor. (Courtesy of Dr. John D. Wright.)

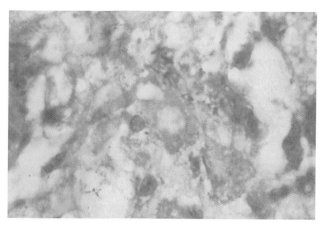

Figure 4-54. Histopathology showing periodic acid–Schiff-positive diastase-resistant intracytoplasmic structures in the tumor cells (periodic acid–Schiff, original magnification × 300). (Courtesy of Dr. John D. Wright.)

GRANULAR CELL TUMOR, AMPUTATION NEUROMA, AND MALIGNANT PERIPHERAL NERVE SHEATH TUMOR

Miscellaneous presumed peripheral nerve tumors of the orbit include granular cell tumor, amputation neuroma, malignant peripheral nerve sheath tumor, and paraganglioma (chemodectoma) (1). Examples of the first three are cited here.

Granular cell tumor is a well-circumscribed benign tumor that has clinical and imaging features similar to those of cavernous hemangioma, neurilemoma, and other well-defined orbital tumors. It frequently involves an extraocular muscle. Although it was originally believed to be a myogenic tumor (granular cell myoblastoma), it is now believed to be a tumor of modified Schwann cell origin. As with other circumscribed orbital tumors, management is complete surgical excision to prevent local recurrence (2).

Amputation neuroma is a benign neural mass that develops following trauma or surgery in which orbital peripheral nerves have been severed. It is prone to occur in the anophthalmic orbit following enucleation. It sometimes is associated with pain. Complete excision is the management of choice (3).

Malignant peripheral nerve sheath tumor (neurofibrosarcoma, malignant schwannoma) is an aggressive neoplasm that apparently arises from Schwann cells or fibroblasts or combinations of the two. Most arise *de novo*, without prior evidence of a benign neurofibroma or neurilemoma. It tends to be invasive, with a high incidence of recurrence after attempted excision. It can infiltrate the superior orbital fissure into the central nervous system. Histopathologically, it is composed of anaplastic spindle or epithelioid cells. Immunohistochemistry and electron microscopy may be required to confirm the diagnosis. Wide surgical excision is the treatment of choice (4).

SELECTED REFERENCES

1. Shields JA. *Diagnosis and management of orbital tumors.* Philadelphia: WB Saunders, 1989:149–152.
2. Jaeger MJ, Green WR, Miller NR, Harris G. Granular cell tumor of the orbit and ocular adnexae. *Surv Ophthalmol* 1987;31:417–423.
3. Messmer EP, Camara J, Boniuk M, Font RL. Amputation neuroma of the orbit. Report of two cases and review of the literature. *Ophthalmology* 1984;91:1420–1423.
4. Jakobiec FA, Font RL, Zimmerman LE. Malignant peripheral nerve sheath tumors of the orbit. A clinicopathologic study of 8 cases. *Trans Am Ophthalmol Soc* 1985;83:17–35.

Granular Cell Tumor, Amputation Neuroma, and Malignant Peripheral Nerve Sheath Tumor

Figs. 4-57 and 4-58 courtesy of Dr. Ramon Font. From Messmer EP, Camara J, Boniuk M, Font RL. Amputation neuroma of the orbit. Report of two cases and review of the literature. *Ophthalmology* 1984;91:1420–1423.

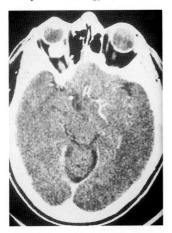

Figure 4-55. Granular cell tumor. Axial computed tomography of a 42-year-old woman who presented with slight pain and diplopia without proptosis. The circumscribed orbital mass, located inferior to the optic nerve, proved to be a granular cell tumor. (Courtesy of Dr. Alan Friedman.)

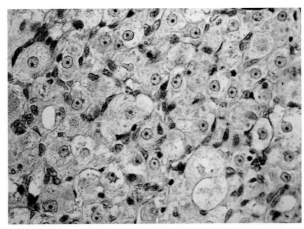

Figure 4-56. Histopathology of granular cell tumor (hematoxylin–eosin, original magnification × 200). (Courtesy of Armed Forces Institute of Pathology, Washington, DC.)

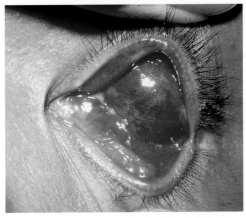

Figure 4-57. Amputation neuroma. Orbital mass in the anophthalmic socket of a 32-year-old man who underwent enucleation at age 7 years for a blind, phthisical eye of uncertain etiology. There is a cystic area above and a solid area below.

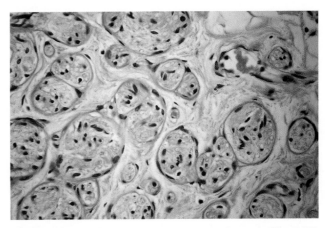

Figure 4-58. Histopathology of the case shown in Fig. 4-57. Note the proliferating nerve bundles surrounded by a perineural sheath and embedded in dense connective tissue, consistent with amputation neuroma.

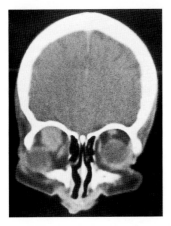

Figure 4-59. Malignant peripheral nerve sheath tumor. Coronal computed tomography showing superior orbital mass in the right orbit of a 79-year-old woman. She had three recurrences and eventually died from brain invasion through the orbital roof.

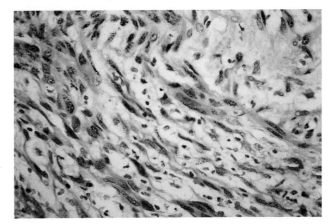

Figure 4-60. Histopathology of malignant peripheral-nerve sheath tumor of the orbit showing malignant spindle and epithelioid cells (hematoxylin–eosin, original magnification × 200).

CHAPTER 5

Optic Nerve, Meningeal, and Other Neural Tumors

JUVENILE PILOCYTIC ASTROCYTOMA (OPTIC NERVE GLIOMA)

Juvenile pilocytic astrocytoma is the most important optic nerve tumor of childhood (1–3). It has distinctive clinical, radiologic, and histopathologic features. Clinically, it generally is diagnosed in the first or second decade of life when the child presents with progressive visual loss and axial proptosis without inflammatory signs. It occasionally becomes clinically apparent in adulthood (4). Because there is perhaps a 40% to 50% incidence of neurofibromatosis associated with this tumor, the affected child should be evaluated for signs of von Recklinghausen's disease, such as cutaneous pigmented macules (*café au lait* spots) and Lisch nodules on the iris. In the early stages, fundus examination may show a swollen optic disc, which later may become pale with the appearance of a retinochoroidal shunt vessel on the margin of the disc (1). The chronic disc edema rarely can induce a choroidal neovascular membrane (5). Computed tomography and magnetic resonance imaging typically show an ovoid mass corresponding to an enlarged optic nerve. A characteristic kink in the midportion of the tumor is often present. Extension into the optic foramen to the chiasm and brain often is present and is seen best with gadolinium-enhanced magnetic resonance imaging. Although it is typically a disease of childhood, in some instances a benign astrocytoma of the optic nerve can occur in adulthood.

Gross pathology shows a optic nerve mass that typically is surrounded by the dura mater. Juvenile pilocytic astrocytoma has typical histopathologic characteristics (1,3). It is composed of a solid proliferation of benign pilocytic astrocytes, sometimes with areas of mucinous degeneration, hemorrhage, and Rosenthal fibers (1,3).

The management of juvenile pilocytic astrocytoma of the optic nerve is complex and controversial. Because the lesion is benign, most authorities prefer to be as conservative as possible. Biopsy generally is contraindicated, because the diagnosis usually can be made with the characteristic clinical and radiographic findings. Asymptomatic lesions often are followed initially without treatment. Serial examinations should be done for pupillary reaction, visual acuity, visual fields, and color vision of both eyes. Most tumors that are confined to the orbit remain relatively stable, but slow growth occasionally can occur. If the patient is blind and has unacceptable proptosis of the affected eye, then complete removal of the mass by lateral orbitotomy is warranted. It usually is not necessary to remove the blind eye in such cases. Progressive lesions that involve the chiasm and brain are sometimes fatal and may require radiotherapy. The role of chemotherapy is uncertain. When the tumor is initially confined to the optic nerve, the mortality is less than 5%. When the hypothalamus is involved, mortality rises to over 50% (2).

SELECTED REFERENCES

1. Shields JA. *Diagnosis and management of orbital tumors.* Philadelphia: WB Saunders, 1989:170–179.
2. Dutton JJ. Gliomas of the anterior visual pathway. *Surv Ophthalmol* 1994;38:427–452.
3. Rao NA, Spencer WH. Optic nerve. In: Spencer WH, ed. *Ophthalmic pathology. An atlas and textbook*, 4th ed, vol 1. Philadelphia: WB Saunders, 1996:596–607.
4. Wulc AE, Bergin DJ, Barnes D, Scaravilli F, Wright JE, McDonald WI. Orbital optic nerve glioma in adult life. *Arch Ophthalmol* 1989;107:1013–1016.
5. Shields JA, Shields CL, De Potter P, Milner RS. Choroidal neovascular membrane as a presenting feature of optic nerve glioma. *Retina* 1997;17:349–350.

Juvenile Pilocytic Astrocytoma of the Optic Nerve

Juvenile pilocytic astrocytoma of the optic nerve has typical clinical and computed tomography features. When it is confined to the orbit and produces a blind eye with progressive irreversible proptosis, the tumor can be removed by a lateral orbitotomy or by a transcranial approach, depending on the extent of the involvement. A clinico-pathologic correlation is shown.

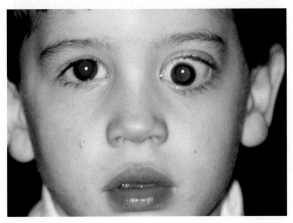

Figure 5-1. Axial proptosis of the left eye in a 4-year-old boy. The proptosis had been progressive for more than 1 year.

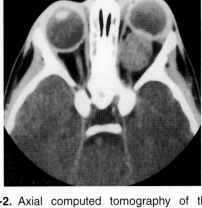

Figure 5-2. Axial computed tomography of the patient shown in Fig. 5-1 revealing a characteristic, well-defined, ovoid mass affecting the optic nerve. The lesion had shown considerable enlargement when compared to a computed tomogram done 1 year earlier.

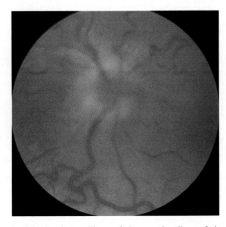

Figure 5-3. Marked swelling of the optic disc of the left eye.

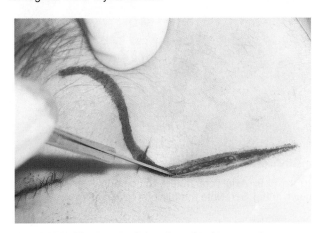

Figure 5-4. The proptosis continued to increase to an unacceptable degree, and surgical excision was elected. The planned skin incision for a superolateral orbitotomy is shown.

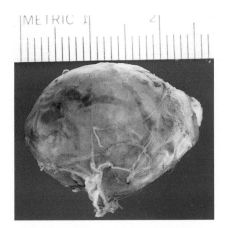

Figure 5-5. Gross appearance of the well-circumscribed mass immediately after surgical removal.

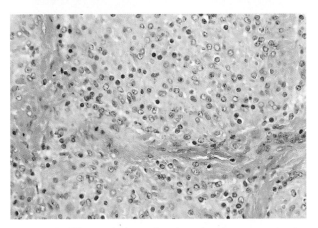

Figure 5-6. Histopathology showing closely compact astrocytes (hematoxylin–eosin, original magnification × 100).

Juvenile pilocytic astrocytoma of the optic nerve has characteristic features with magnetic resonance imaging. When the proptosis is more advanced, the proptosis converts from an axial direction to a down and out direction, conforming to the contour of the bony orbit.

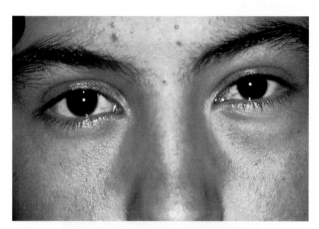

Figure 5-7. Proptosis of the left eye in a 15-year-old boy.

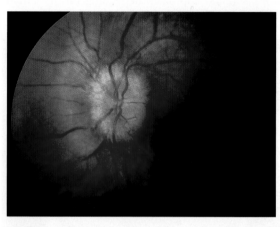

Figure 5-8. Hyperemia and edema of the optic disc in the patient shown in Fig. 5-7.

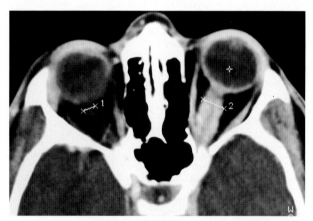

Figure 5-9. Axial computed tomography of the patient shown in Fig. 5-7. Note the fusiform lesion of the optic nerve.

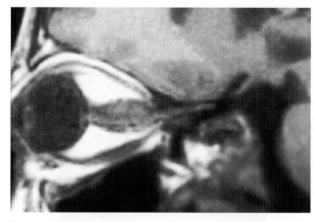

Figure 5-10. Sagittal magnetic resonance imaging in T1-weighted image showing the same lesion shown in Fig. 5-9.

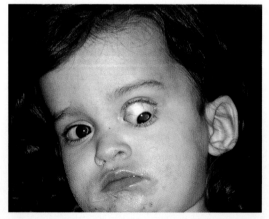

Figure 5-11. Proptosis and downward displacement of the left eye secondary to a juvenile pilocytic astrocytoma in a 2-year-old girl. The eye was blind, and the progressive proptosis prompted surgical removal of the tumor.

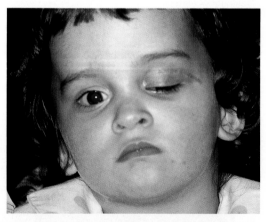

Figure 5-12. Appearance of the child shown in Fig. 5-11, 3 months after removal of the tumor. There is no more proptosis, and the blepharoptosis is to be corrected when the child is older.

Fundus Changes with Juvenile Pilocytic Astrocytoma of the Optic Nerve

The most common fundus changes with juvenile pilocytic astrocytoma of the optic nerve are a swollen optic disc followed by a retinochoroidal shunt vessel and pallor of the optic disc. The venous stasis secondary to optic disc involvement can prompt development of a juxtapapillary choroidal neovascular membrane.

Figs. 5-16 through 5-18 from Shields JA, Shields CL, De Potter P, Milner RS. Choroidal neovascular membrane as a presenting feature of optic nerve glioma. *Retina* 1997;17:349–350.

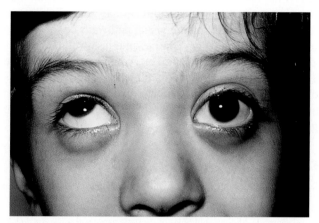

Figure 5-13. Proptosis of the left eye and inability of upgaze secondary to a juvenile pilocytic astrocytoma of the optic nerve in a 6-year-old boy.

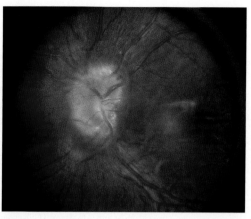

Figure 5-14. Swelling and hyperemia of the optic disc in the child shown in Fig. 5-13. Note the retinochoroidal shunt vessel on the superotemporal margin of the optic disc.

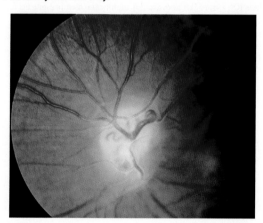

Figure 5-15. Appearance of the same optic disc 4 years later. Note the optic disc pallor and distinct retinochoroidal shunt vessel.

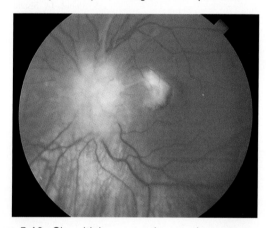

Figure 5-16. Choroidal neovascular membrane temporal to chronically swollen optic disc in a 16-year-old girl. The cause of the optic disc changes and neovascular membrane was not initially determined.

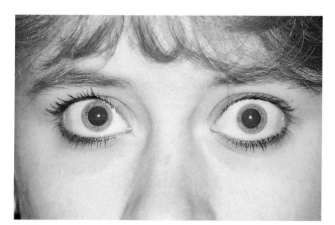

Figure 5-17. A few weeks later, the patient shown in Fig. 5-16 was realized to have proptosis of the left eye, which prompted orbital computed tomography.

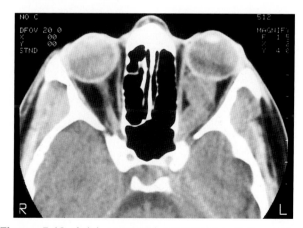

Figure 5-18. Axial computed tomography of the patient shown in Fig. 5-16 demonstrating the characteristic findings of a juvenile pilocytic astrocytoma of the optic nerve. Note the characteristic kink in the midportion of the nerve nasally.

MALIGNANT OPTIC NERVE ASTROCYTOMA

The benign pilocytic astrocytoma usually has its clinical onset in childhood. There is also a malignant form of optic nerve astrocytoma that occurs in adulthood and which usually is not associated with neurofibromatosis (1–5). The patient characteristically presents with acute onset of progressive visual loss in one eye associated with a variety of oculomotor palsies. If the optic disc is involved, fundus examination may disclose a hemorrhagic, edematous optic disc with central retinal vein obstruction. Imaging studies may show a diffuse mass involving the visual pathways or sometimes a circumscribed, round to ovoid orbital mass, which can become less well defined as it progresses. The tumor rapidly can invade the central nervous system and cause death. Histopathologically, it is composed of areas of anaplastic fibrillary astrocytes with pleomorphism and mitotic figures. The best treatment appears to be prompt and wide surgical excision, often via transcranial route. Orbital exenteration also may be necessary. The prognosis is guarded.

SELECTED REFERENCES

1. Hoyt WF, Meshel LG, Lessell S, Schatz NJ, Suckling RD. Malignant optic glioma of adulthood. *Brain* 1973;96:121–132.
2. Harper CG, Stewart-Wynne EG. Malignant optic gliomas in adults. *Arch Neurol* 1978;35:731–735.
3. Spoor TC, Kennerdell JS, Martinez AJ, Zorub D. Malignant gliomas of the optic nerve pathways. *Am J Ophthalmol* 1980;89:284–292.
4. Rudd A, Rees JE, Kennedy P, Weller RO, Blackwood W. Malignant optic nerve gliomas in adults. *J Clin Neuro-ophthalmol* 1985;5:238–243.
5. Shields JA, Shields CL, De Potter P, Milner RS. Choroidal neovascular membrane as a presenting feature of optic nerve glioma. *Retina* 1997;17:349–350.

Malignant Optic Nerve Astrocytoma

Malignant glioma of the visual pathways can cause rapid visual loss, oculomotor palsies, and retinal vascular obstruction.

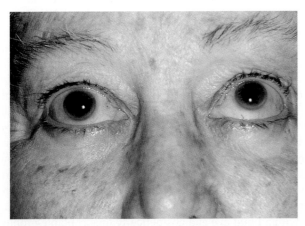

Figure 5-19. Paresis of upgaze of the right eye in a 78-year-old woman. (Courtesy of Drs. Jurji Bilyk and Peter Savino.)

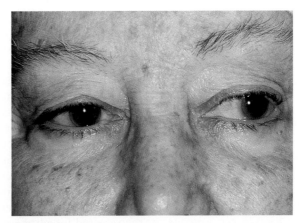

Figure 5-20. Paresis of adduction of the right eye in the same patient. (Courtesy of Drs. Jurji Bilyk and Peter Savino.)

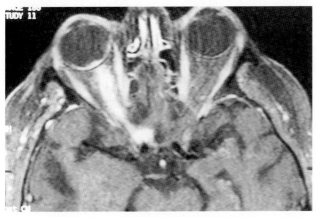

Figure 5-21. Axial magnetic resonance imaging in T1-weighted image of the patient shown in Fig. 5-19 demonstrating a diffuse enhancing mass involving the optic nerve to the optic chiasm. (Courtesy of Drs. Jurji Bilyk and Peter Savino.)

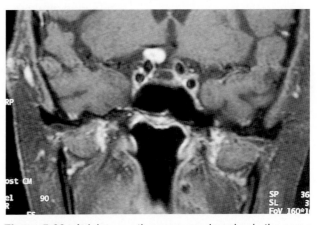

Figure 5-22. Axial magnetic resonance imaging in the same patient demonstrating an enhancing mass in the optic chiasm. (Courtesy of Drs. Jurji Bilyk and Peter Savino.)

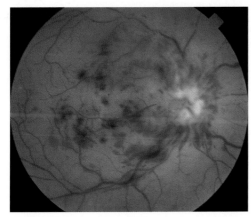

Figure 5-23. Fundus photograph showing optic disc edema, vascular congestion, and hemorrhage in a 52-year-old man with malignant optic nerve glioma. (Courtesy of Dr. Lee Jampol.)

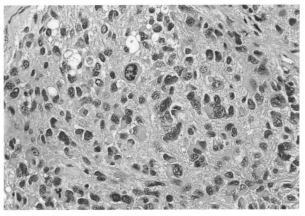

Figure 5-24. Histopathology of malignant optic nerve astrocytoma showing malignant glial cells (hematoxylin–eosin, original magnification × 150). (Courtesy of Dr. Ralph C. Eagle Jr.)

MENINGIOMA

Meningioma is a benign neoplasm that arises from the arachnoid layer of the meninges (1–4). Although there are several types and locations, the most important with regard to the orbit are the primary optic nerve sheath meningioma and the sphenoid wing meningioma. Primary optic nerve sheath meningioma arises from the arachnoid cells that surround the optic nerve. It appears to have a biphasic age distribution, with those that occur in childhood being somewhat more aggressive and those of adulthood being less aggressive (2).

Both optic nerve sheath meningioma and sphenoid wing meningioma seem to be more common in middle-aged women. The affected patient generally presents with visual loss and a swollen or atrophic optic disc, often with a characteristic retinochoroidal shunt vessel at the optic disc margin. Later, there is slowly progressive proptosis of the affected eye. The lesion occasionally can be bilateral. When it is confined to the optic canal, it can produce signs of optic neuritis and the diagnosis may be more difficult. Imaging studies show an enlarged optic nerve with either a fusiform or round configuration. Because surgical excision invariably leads to blindness, conservative management generally is recommended with surgical excision being reserved for advanced tumors with a blind eye and cosmetically unacceptable proptosis. Although surgical removal of the tumor with an attempt to spare the optic nerve has been performed (5), patients treated in that manner are very likely to develop severe optic atrophy and blindness. Irradiation may provide benefit in some cases. This benign tumor has an excellent systemic prognosis (4).

Sphenoid wing meningioma can produce somewhat different symptoms and signs than the optic nerve sheath meningioma. The patient is generally a middle-aged woman who initially develops slowly progressive proptosis and swelling of the temporal fossa, followed later by visual impairment as the neoplasm encroaches upon the optic canal. Needle biopsy has been employed to make the diagnosis of both optic nerve sheath meningioma and sphenoid wing meningioma in selected cases (1,6). Surgical excision can be considered with collaboration between an ophthalmologist and neurosurgeon if vision is threatened or if there is progressive disease. Chemotherapy and radiotherapy also are options for progressive disease with visual loss.

SELECTED REFERENCES

1. Shields JA. *Diagnosis and management of orbital tumors.* Philadelphia: WB Saunders, 1989:180–186.
2. Karp LA, Zimmerman LE, Borit A, Spencer W. Primary intraorbital meningiomas. *Arch Ophthalmol* 1974; 91:24–28.
3. Wright JE, Call NB, Liaricos S. Primary optic nerve meningioma. *Br J Ophthalmol* 1980;64:553–558.
4. Dutton JJ. Optic nerve sheath meningiomas. *Surv Ophthalmol* 1992;37:167–183.
5. Mark LE, Kennerdell JS, Maroon JC, Rosenbaum A, Heinz R, Johnson BL. Microsurgical removal of a primary intraorbital meningioma. *Am J Ophthalmol* 1978;86:704–709.
6. Kennerdell JS, Dubois PJ, Dekker A, Johnson BL. CT-guided fine needle aspiration biopsy of orbital optic nerve tumors. *Ophthalmology* 1980;87:491–496.

Primary Optic Nerve Sheath Meningioma

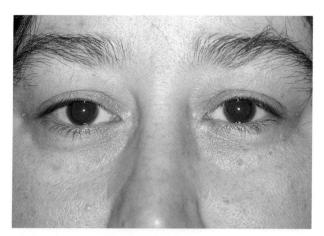

Figure 5-25. Minimal prominence of the right eye in a 38-year-old woman with mild visual loss.

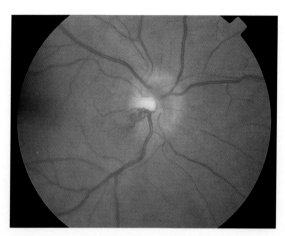

Figure 5-26. Appearance of the optic disc in the patient shown in Fig. 5-25 demonstrating retinochoroidal shunt vessel on the inferotemporal margin of the optic disc. Photographs taken 2 years early showed no shunt vessel, which was observed to develop gradually.

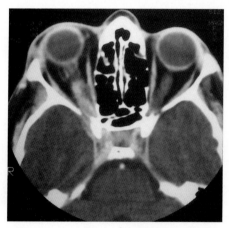

Figure 5-27. Axial computed tomography showing meningioma of the right optic nerve sheath.

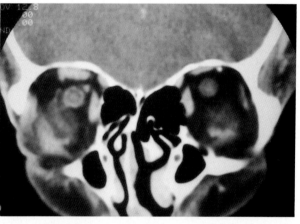

Figure 5-28. Coronal computed tomography showing the same lesion depicted in Fig. 5-27.

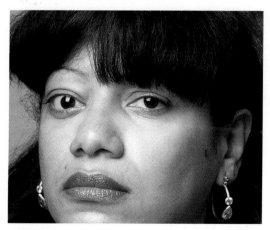

Figure 5-29. Proptosis of the right eye in a 39-year-old woman with an optic nerve sheath meningioma.

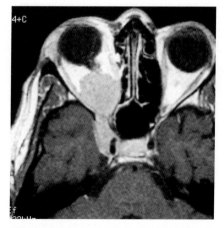

Figure 5-30. Coronal magnetic resonance imaging in T1-weighted image of the patient shown in Fig. 5-29 revealing a round mass arising from the posterior aspect of the optic nerve with extension through the optic canal into the chiasm. The tumor was resected via a transcranial route.

Aggressive Optic Nerve Sheath Meningioma

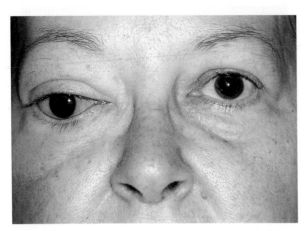

Figure 5-31. Appearance of the patient who underwent enucleation elsewhere several years earlier for a blind, uncomfortable eye. She was referred because of recent inability to retain the prosthesis.

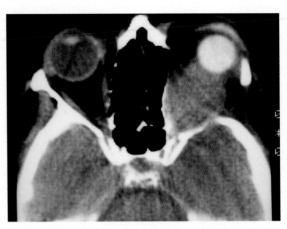

Figure 5-32. Axial computed tomography of the patient shown in Fig. 5-31 demonstrating an orbital mass posterior to the ball implant. Such a patient would be a good candidate for diagnostic orbital fine-needle aspiration biopsy.

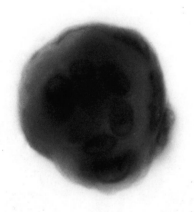

Figure 5-33. Cytology of fine-needle aspiration biopsy of optic nerve sheath meningioma showing a whorl of meningothelial cells. (Papanicolaou, original magnification × 250).

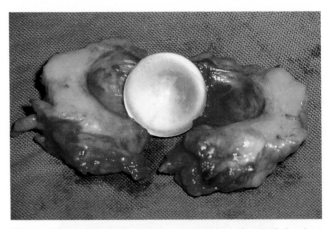

Figure 5-34. Surgical specimen showing the ball implant surrounded by dense fleshy tumor tissue. Histopathology confirmed the diagnosis of meningioma.

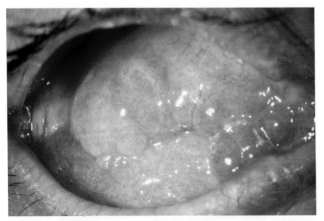

Figure 5-35. Appearance of the socket 3 years later showing recurrence of fleshy tumor tissue filling the palpebral fissure.

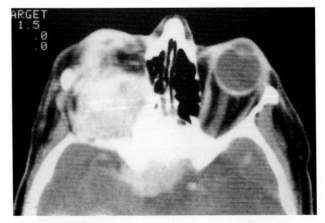

Figure 5-36. Axial computed tomography performed at the same time as Fig. 5-35 demonstrating massive recurrence of the meningioma involving the orbit and intracranial tissues. The tumor was treated successfully by a combined intracranial approach and orbital exenteration.

Sphenoid Wing Meningioma with Orbital Involvement

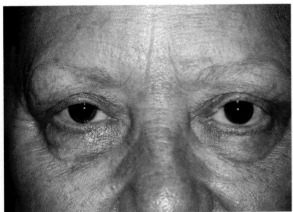

Figure 5-37. Proptosis of the left eye in a 63-year-old woman.

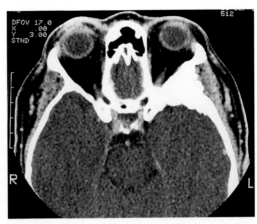

Figure 5-38. Axial computed tomography of the patient shown in Fig. 5-37 demonstrating hyperostosis of the greater wing of the sphenoid on the left side, a finding characteristic of meningioma.

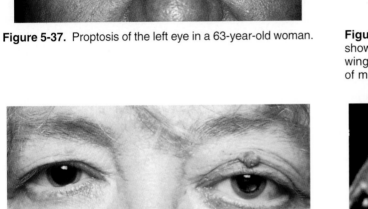

Figure 5-39. Proptosis and blepharoptosis of the left eye in a 54-year-old woman.

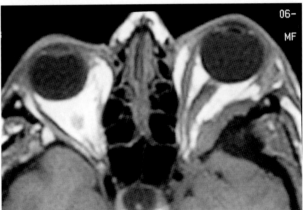

Figure 5-40. Axial magnetic resonance imaging in T1-weighted image of the patient shown in Fig. 5-39. Note the hyperostosis and the soft-tissue component of the tumor in the orbit.

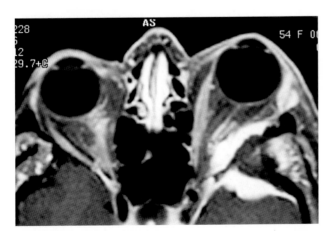

Figure 5-41. Axial magnetic resonance imaging in T1-weighted image with gadolinium enhancement showing marked enhancement of the soft-tissue component of the placoid tumor in the orbit, brain, and temporal fossa. Magnetic resonance imaging is superior to computed tomography for defining the extent of soft-tissue involvement.

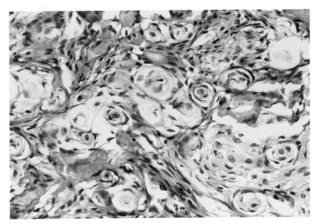

Figure 5-42. Histopathology of orbital meningioma showing characteristic whorls of meningothelial cells (hematoxylin–eosin, original magnification × 100).

PRIMITIVE NEUROECTODERMAL TUMOR AND PRIMARY ORBITAL NEUROBLASTOMA

Other neural tumors of the orbit that are not discussed in other sections include neuroepithelial tumors, such as primary orbital neuroblastoma and primitive neuroectodermal tumor. These are closely related tumors that have been reported in the literature as separate entities (1–5). Other closely related tumors, such as granular cell tumor, esthesioneuroblastoma, paraganglioma (chemodectoma), and primary orbital melanoma, are discussed in other chapters or in other textbooks (4).

Primitive neuroectodermal tumor is a neural tumor of childhood that is being recognized more frequently. It is estimated to represent 4% to 17% of all pediatric soft-tissue tumors and is being recognized more frequently, having been called sarcoma in the past (1). It has many clinical and histopathologic features similar to those of neuroblastoma and Ewing's tumor, and its differentiation from these and other pediatric orbital tumors has been discussed. Clinically, it presents as rapid proptosis and displacement of the eye in an adolescent or young adult. Imaging studies may show an invasive mass with bone destruction (1). Management is similar to that of rhabdomyosarcoma. A biopsy should be done, removing as much tumor tissue as possible, followed by chemotherapy and possibly irradiation, preferably under the direction of a pediatric oncologist and radiation oncologist.

The best known neuroblastoma of the orbit is metastatic neuroblastoma from the adrenal gland. However, in rare instances, primary orbital neuroblastoma has been diagnosed in the orbit (2,3). In contrast to primitive neuroectodermal tumor, it seems to be more common in adults. It begins as a circumscribed tumor, which later becomes more invasive. Management is surgical resection, often combined with chemotherapy and irradiation.

SELECTED REFERENCES

1. Singh AD, Husson M, Shields CL, De Potter P, Shields JA. Primitive neuroectodermal tumor of the orbit. *Arch Ophthalmol* 1994;112:217–221.
2. Jakobiec FA, Klepach GL, Crissman JD, Spoor TC. Primary differentiated neuroblastoma of the orbit. *Ophthalmology* 1987;94:255–266.
3. Bullock JD, Goldberg SH, Rakes SM, Felder DS, Connelly PJ. Primary orbital neuroblastoma. *Arch Ophthalmol* 1989;107:1031–1033.
4. Shields JA. *Diagnosis and management of orbital tumors*. Philadelphia: WB Saunders, 1989:165–166.
5. Rootman J, Robertson WD. Neuroepithelial tumors. In: Rootman J, ed. *Diseases of the orbit*. Philadelphia: JB Lippincott Co., 1988:329–334.

Primitive Neuroectodermal Tumor and Primary Orbital Neuroblastoma

Figs. 5-43 through 5-45 from Singh AD, Husson M, Shields CL, De Potter P, Shields JA. Primitive neuroectodermal tumor of the orbit. *Arch Ophthalmol* 1994;112:217–221.

Figs. 5-46 through 5-48 courtesy of Dr. Frederick Jakobiec. From Jakobiec FA, Klepach GL, Crissman JD, Spoor TC. Primary differentiated neuroblastoma of the orbit. *Ophthalmology* 1987;94:255–266.

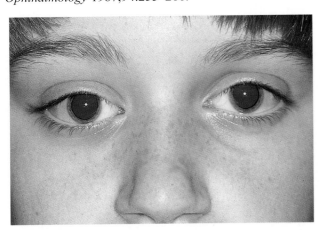

Figure 5-43. Primitive neuroectodermal tumor. Proptosis of the right eye in a 10-year-old girl.

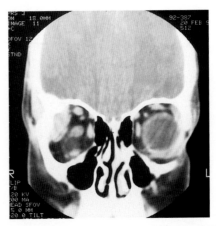

Figure 5-44. Coronal computed tomography of the patient shown in Figure 5-43 demonstrating a superotemporal orbital tumor with bone erosion and hyperostosis.

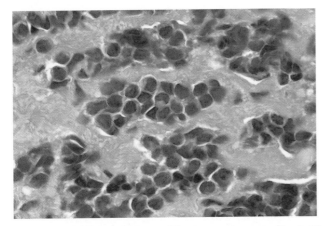

Figure 5-45. Histopathology of the tumor shown in Fig. 5-43 revealing nests of neuroblastic cells in a fibrous tissue stroma.

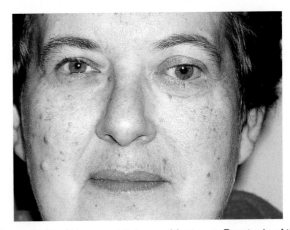

Figure 5-46. Primary orbital neuroblastoma. Proptosis of the left eye in a middle-aged woman.

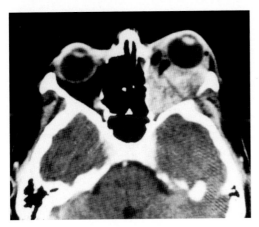

Figure 5-47. Axial computed tomography of the woman shown in Fig. 5-46 demonstrating a large irregular mass filling most of the orbit.

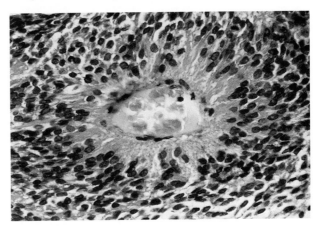

Figure 5-48. Histopathology of the lesion shown in Fig. 5-47 demonstrating neuroblastic cells with a neuroblastic rosette (hematoxylin–eosin, original magnification × 200).

CHAPTER 6

Myogenic Tumors

RHABDOMYOSARCOMA

Rhabdomyosarcoma is the most common primary orbital malignancy of childhood (1–5). In the authors' series, it accounted for only 1% of biopsied orbital masses (2) and 4% of all biopsied orbital masses in children (3). Orbital rhabdomyosarcoma generally occurs in the first two decades of life with rapidly progressive proptosis and displacement of the eye (1–10). The tumor can arise primarily in the orbit, or it can arise in the sinuses or nasal cavity and secondarily extend to involve the orbit. The most characteristic presenting features of orbital rhabdomyosarcoma is a rapid onset and progression of proptosis, conjunctival chemosis, and displacement of the globe. It occasionally can occur as an epibulbar mass without deep orbital involvement. Orbital rhabdomyosarcoma has been observed many years after orbital irradiation for retinoblastoma (10).

Computed tomography demonstrates a large moderately well-circumscribed but irregular orbital mass, which may extend to involve the adjacent orbital bones or sinuses. Magnetic resonance imaging demonstrates an irregular mass that enhances with contrast material.

Orbital rhabdomyosarcoma probably arises from primitive pleuripotential mesenchymal cells with a propensity to differentiate toward skeletal muscle. Several histologic variations of rhabdomyosarcoma occur in the orbit. The embryonal type is most common, whereas the alveolar type appears to be the most malignant (5,6). Orbital rhabdomyosarcoma should be managed by a prompt biopsy with histopathologic confirmation of the diagnosis, followed by radiotherapy and chemotherapy (7). Using this modern regimen, the survival rate has increased dramatically in recent years (8).

SELECTED REFERENCES

1. Shields JA. *Diagnosis and management of orbital tumors.* Philadelphia: WB Saunders, 1989:244–252.
2. Shields JA, Bakewell B, Augsburger JJ, Flanagan JC. Classification and incidence of space-occupying lesions of the orbit. A survey of 645 biopsies. *Arch Ophthalmol* 1984;102:1606–1611.
3. Shields JA, Bakewell B, Augsburger JJ, Donoso LA, Bernardino V. Space-occupying orbital masses in children: a review of 250 consecutive biopsies. *Ophthalmology* 1986;93:379–384.
4. Shields JA. Rhabdomyosarcoma of the orbit. In: Hornblass A, ed. *Ophthalmic plastic and reconstructive surgery.* Baltimore: Williams & Wilkins, 1987;980–985.
5. Jakobiec FA, Font RL. Orbit. In: Spencer WH, Font RL, Green WR, Howes EL Jr, Jakobiec FA, Zimmerman LE, eds. *Ophthalmic pathology. An atlas and textbook.* 4th ed. Philadelphia: WB Saunders Co., 1996: 2556–2560.
6. Knowles DM II, Jakobiec FA, Potter GD, Jones IS. Ophthalmic striated muscle neoplasms. *Surv Ophthalmol* 1976;21:219–261.
7. Abramson DH, Ellsworth RM, Tretter P, Wolff JA, Kitchin FD. The treatment of orbital rhabdomyosarcoma with irradiation and chemotherapy. *Ophthalmology* 1979;86:1330–1335.
8. Wharam M, Beltangady M, Hays D, Heyn R, Rabab A, Soule E, Tefft M, Maurer H. Localized orbital rhabdomyosarcoma. An interim report of the intergroup rhabdomyosarcoma study committee. *Ophthalmology* 1987;94:251–254.
9. Shields CL, Shields JA. Orbital rhabdomyosarcoma. In: Fraunfelder FT, Roy H, eds. *Current ocular therapy,* 5th ed. Philadelphia: WB Saunders, 1999 (*in press*).
10. Wilson MC, Shields JA, Shields CL, Litzky L. Orbital rhabdomyosarcoma fifty seven years after radiotherapy for retinoblastoma. *Orbit* 1996;15:97–100.

Orbital Rhabdomyosarcoma

Orbital rhabdomyosarcoma usually has characteristic clinical features, imaging studies, and histopathology. A typical case with clinicopathologic correlation is shown.

From Shields JA, Shields CL, Eagle RC Jr, Nowinski T. Orbital rhabdomyosarcoma. *Arch Ophthalmol* 1987;105:700–701.

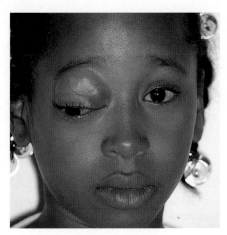

Figure 6-1. Proptosis and downward displacement of the right eye by a superior orbital mass in a 12-year-old girl.

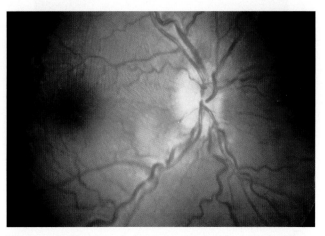

Figure 6-2. Fundus photograph of the right eye showing a slightly swollen optic disc and tortuous retinal veins secondary to compression of the globe by an orbital mass.

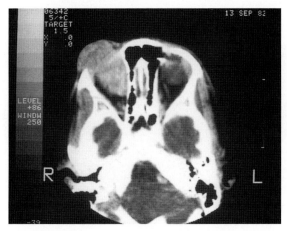

Figure 6-3. Axial computed tomography showing a superonasal orbital mass.

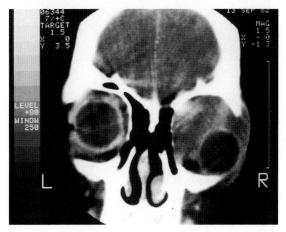

Figure 6-4. Coronal computed tomography showing extent of the lesion. Coronal computed tomography is important in planning the best surgical approach to biopsy.

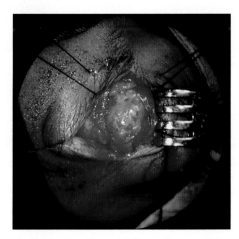

Figure 6-5. Exposure of tumor through a superonasal cutaneous approach.

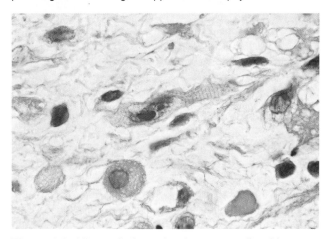

Figure 6-6. Histopathology showing strap cells with cross-striations (hematoxylin–eosin, original magnification × 200).

If not treated promptly, orbital rhabdomyosarcoma can show rapid progression. An example of a cavitary rhabdomyosarcoma that initially simulated a lymphangioma is illustrated.

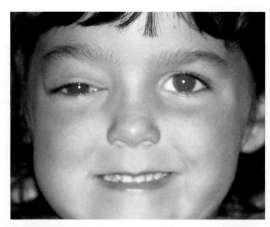

Figure 6-7. Blepharoptosis, proptosis, and downward displacement of the right eye in a 4-year-old girl.

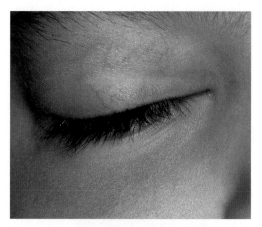

Figure 6-8. Closer view of the right eye. A biopsy was not done because the clinical findings and magnetic resonance imaging (shown in Figs. 6-11 and 6-12) suggested the diagnosis of lymphangioma.

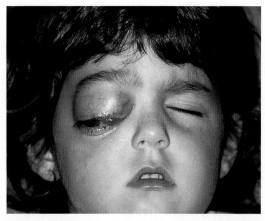

Figure 6-9. Appearance of the patient 10 days later showing rapid progression of proptosis and conjunctival chemosis.

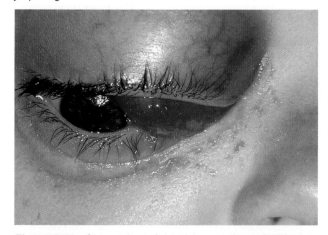

Figure 6-10. Closer view of the right eye shown in Fig. 6-9.

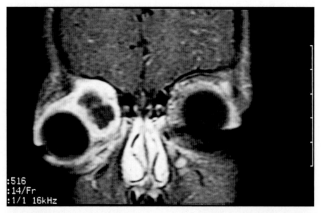

Figure 6-11. Coronal magnetic resonance imaging in T1-weighted imaged with gadolinium enhancement. Note the nonenhancing central area compatible with blood. This accounted for the original diagnosis of lymphangioma with hemorrhage.

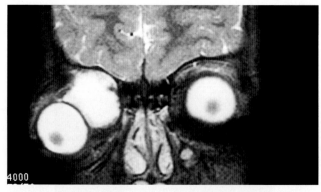

Figure 6-12. Coronal magnetic resonance imaging in T2-weighted image showing extent of the lesion with central cavity suggestive of blood or proteinaceous material.

Orbital Rhabdomyosarcoma—Biopsy Approach

In planning a biopsy of orbital rhabdomyosarcoma, it is important to obtain good axial and coronal imaging studies with computed tomography or magnetic resonance imaging. The approach to biopsy should be determined based on those studies. The goal of surgery is to remove as much of the lesion as possible without damaging vital structures such as the optic nerve and extraocular muscles. A case is illustrated.

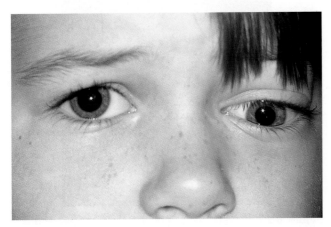

Figure 6-13. Proptosis and downward displacement of the left eye in a 4-year-old girl.

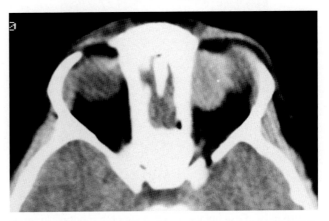

Figure 6-14. Axial computed tomography showing a superonasal ovoid orbital mass.

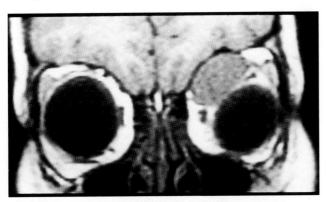

Figure 6-15. Coronal magnetic resonance imaging in T1-weighted image showing superonasal mass with downward displacement of the globe.

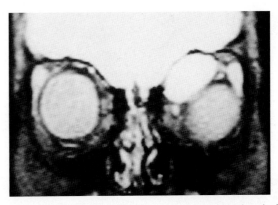

Figure 6-16. Coronal magnetic resonance imaging in T2-weighted image showing mass.

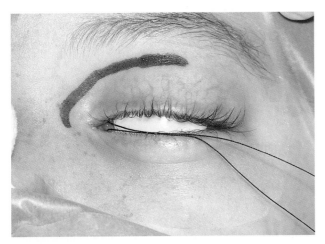

Figure 6-17. Outline of the planned superonasal eyelid crease incision based on review of the imaging studies.

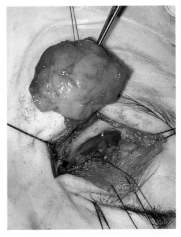

Figure 6-18. View after surgical excision showing intact tumor (*top*). There was no apparent residual tumor in the orbit.

Epibulbar Rhabdomyosarcoma without Proptosis

In some instances, rhabdomyosarcoma can occur in the anterior orbit, conjunctiva, or eyelid. A case is illustrated. In such instances, it may be possible to entirely remove the tumor. It is still not known whether such patients should be treated with additional irradiation and/or chemotherapy but, in most cases, such supplementary treatment has been recommended because of the malignant nature of the tumor.

From Joffe L, Shields JA, Pearah D. Epibulbar rhabdomyosarcoma without proptosis. *J Pediatr Ophthalmol* 1977;14:364–367.

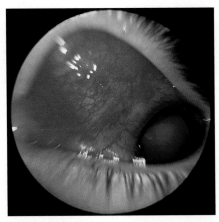

Figure 6-19. Firm epibulbar mass superotemporally in an 8-year-old boy.

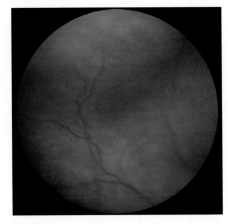

Figure 6-20. Fundus photograph superotemporally showing compression of the globe by the mass. The referring diagnosis was possible choroidal melanoma with extraocular extension.

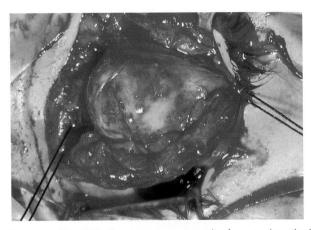

Figure 6-21. Epibulbar mass exposed after conjunctival incision.

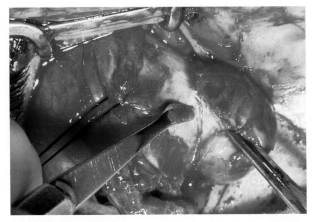

Figure 6-22. Epibulbar mass being removed by shaving excision from the sclera.

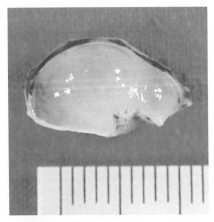

Figure 6-23. Sectioned tumor after removal. The small notch in the capsule represents the site where some tissue was removed postoperatively for possible electron microscopy.

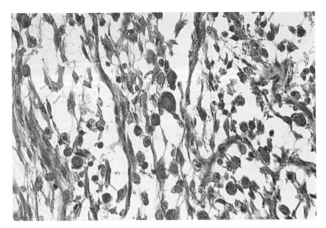

Figure 6-24. Histopathology showing malignant strap cells compatible with rhabdomyosarcoma.

Advanced Orbital Rhabdomyosarcoma

If not treated soon after its clinical onset, orbital rhabdomyosarcoma can rapidly progress to an advanced state. Such advanced cases often require orbital exenteration as well as chemotherapy and irradiation.

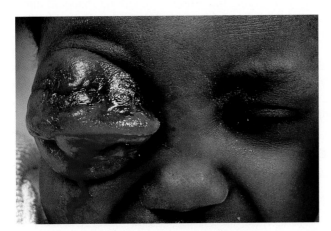

Figure 6-25. Advanced orbital rhabdomyosarcoma in a child from South Africa. (Courtesy of Dr. Ellen Ankor.)

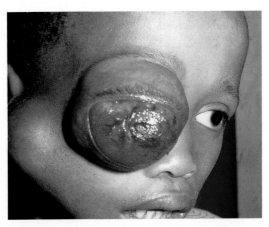

Figure 6-26. Advanced orbital rhabdomyosarcoma with metastasis to preauricular lymph nodes in a child from South Africa. (Courtesy of Dr. Ellen Ankor.)

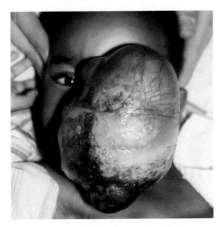

Figure 6-27. Far advanced orbital rhabdomyosarcoma in a child from South Africa. (Courtesy of Dr. Eugene Meyer.)

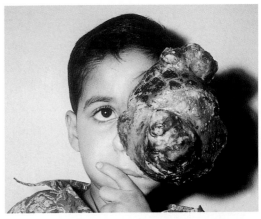

Figure 6-28. Far advanced orbital rhabdomyosarcoma in a child whose parents refused treatment. (Courtesy of Dr. Lorenz Zimmerman and Armed Forces Institute of Pathology, Washington, DC.)

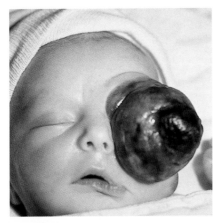

Figure 6-29. Congenital orbital rhabdomyosarcoma present at birth. The child had widespread metastasis at birth and died shortly thereafter. (Courtesy of Dr. Nongnard Chan.)

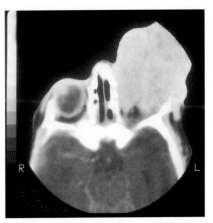

Figure 6-30. Axial computed tomography of the child shown in Fig. 6-29 demonstrating the extent of the orbital tumor. (Courtesy of Dr. Nongnard Chan.)

MALIGNANT RHABDOID TUMOR

Malignant rhabdoid tumors is a neoplasm that occurs in the kidney of infants and young children. Although it originally was described as a "rhabdomyosarcomatoid" variant of Wilm's tumor, it subsequently was recognized as a distinct entity that sometimes can occur in extrarenal sites, including the orbit (1–5). Orbital rhabdoid tumor is an aggressive neoplasm that can occur in children or adults. It has been described in the orbit after enucleation and irradiation for retinoblastoma. It initially is circumscribed, but it can become infiltrative and invade bone. Histopathology reveals a poorly differentiated tumor that shows positive immunoreactivity for vimentin, cytokeratin, and epithelial membrane antigen and negative immunoreactivity for myoglobin, muscle-specific antigen, desmin, and HMB-45. The treatment is surgical excision, chemotherapy, and irradiation, similar to the treatment of rhabdomyosarcoma.

SELECTED REFERENCES

1. Rootman J, Damji KF, Dimmick JE. Malignant rhabdoid tumor of the orbit. *Ophthalmology* 1989;96: 1650–1654.
2. Johnson LN, Sexton FM, Goldberg SH. Poorly differentiated primary orbital sarcoma (presumed malignant rhabdoid tumor). *Arch Ophthalmol* 1991;105:1275–1278.
3. Niffenegger JH, Jakobiec FA, Shore JW, Albert DM. Adult extrarenal rhabdoid tumor of the lacrimal gland. *Ophthalmology* 1992;99:567–574.
4. Walford N, Defarrai R, Slater RM, et al. Intraorbital rhabdoid tumour following bilateral retinoblastoma. *Histopathology* 1992;20:170–173.
5. Gunduz K, Shields JA, Eagle RC Jr, Shields CL, De Potter P, Klombers L. Malignant rhabdoid tumor of the orbit. *Arch Ophthalmol* 1998;116:243–246.

Malignant Rhabdoid Tumor of the Orbit

In young children, malignant rhabdoid can be highly aggressive, with recurrence and extension into the central nervous system. A clinicopathologic correlation is shown.

From Gunduz K, Shields JA, Eagle RC Jr, Shields CL, De Potter P, Klombers L. Malignant rhabdoid tumor of the orbit. *Arch Ophthalmol* 1998;116:243–246.

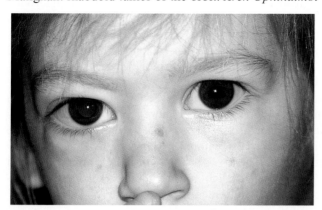

Figure 6-31. Proptosis of the right eye in a 36-month-old girl. The dilated, fixed pupil did not react to light.

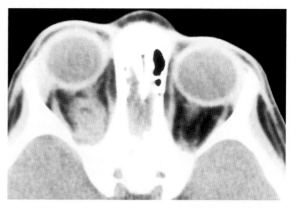

Figure 6-32. Axial computed tomography showing an ovoid mass in muscle cone extending to the orbital apex. Piece-meal excisional biopsy revealed features of rhabdoid tumor. The child was treated with chemotherapy (vincristine and actinomycin D) and radiotherapy (5,000 cGy).

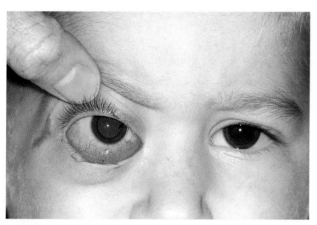

Figure 6-33. About 8 months later, the child presented with recurrent proptosis and conjunctival chemosis.

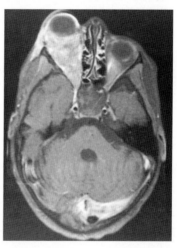

Figure 6-34. Axial magnetic resonance imaging in T1-weighted image showing massive orbital recurrence. Orbital exenteration was performed. A few months later, the tumor recurred in the orbit maxillary sinus and brain, and the child died shortly thereafter.

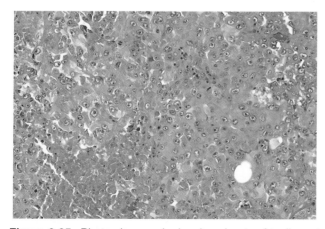

Figure 6-35. Photomicrograph showing sheets of malignant tumor cells (hematoxylin–eosin, original magnification × 50).

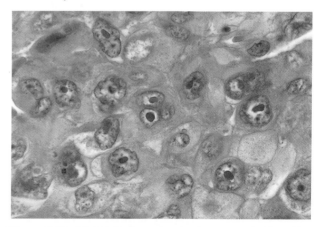

Figure 6-36. Histopathology showing large anaplastic epithelioid cells. Immunohistochemistry and electron microscopy supported the diagnosis of extrarenal rhabdoid tumor (hematoxylin–eosin, original magnification × 250).

LEIOMYOMA AND LEIOMYOSARCOMA

Smooth-muscle tumors in the orbit can be benign (leiomyoma) or malignant (leiomyosarcoma) (1,2). Leiomyoma appears to be a tumor of children and young adults. It produces painless proptosis like most other benign tumors. Imaging studies generally show a well-circumscribed, round to ovoid mass anywhere in the orbit. It is composed of well-differentiated spindle cells (3). The diagnosis can be confirmed with immunohistochemistry, which shows positivity for smooth-muscle antigen. Management is complete surgical excision of the mass.

Leiomyosarcoma is a malignant smooth-muscle tumor. It has a tendency to occur in middle-aged or older women (4–6). It generally has a more rapid onset and progression than leiomyoma. It begins as a circumscribed lesion that may be indistinguishable from other well-defined orbital masses. Histopathology shows more anaplastic spindle cells that also show positive immunoreactivity to smooth-muscle antigen. Orbital leiomyosarcoma is known to occur after irradiation for retinoblastoma (7). The management is wide excision including orbital exenteration if necessary.

SELECTED REFERENCES

1. Shields JA. *Diagnosis and management of orbital tumors.* Philadelphia: WB Saunders, 1989:252–256.
2. Jakobiec FA, Howard GM, Rosen M, et al. Leiomyoma and leiomyosarcoma of the orbit. *Am J Ophthalmol* 1975;80:1028–1042.
3. Sanborn GE, Valenzuela RE, Green WR. Leiomyoma of the orbit. *Am J Ophthalmol* 1979;87:371–375.
4. Meekins BB, Dutton JJ, Proia AD. Primary orbital leiomyosarcoma. A case report and review of the literature. *Arch Ophthalmol* 1988;106;82–86.
5. Wojno T, Tenzel RR, Nadju M. Orbital leiomyosarcoma. *Arch Ophthalmol* 1983;101:1566-1568.
6. Kaltreider SA, Destro M, Lemke BN. Leiomyosarcoma of the orbit. A case report and review of the literature. *Ophthal Plast Reconstr Surg* 1987;3:35–41.
7. Font RL, Jurco S III, Brechner RJ. Postradiation leiomyosarcoma of the orbit complicating bilateral retinoblastoma. *Arch Ophthalmol* 1983;101:1557–1561.

Leiomyoma and Leiomyosarcoma

Figs. 6-40 through 6-42 courtesy of Dr. Alan Proia. From Meekins BB, Dutton JJ, Proia AD. Primary orbital leiomyosarcoma. A case report and review of the literature. *Arch Ophthalmol* 1988;106:82–86.

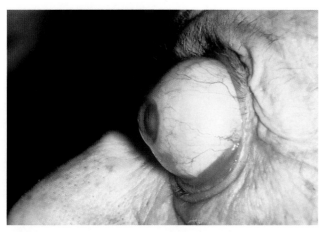

Figure 6-37. Leiomyoma. Marked axial proptosis in an 86-year-old woman. (Courtesy of Dr. John Finlay.)

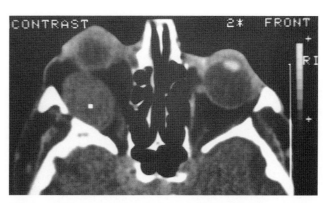

Figure 6-38. Axial computed tomography showing circumscribed, soft-tissue orbital mass. (Courtesy of Dr. John Finlay.)

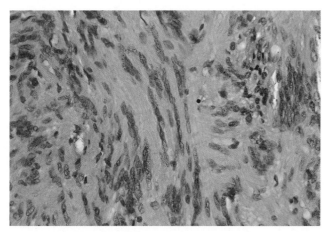

Figure 6-39. Histopathology of the lesion shown in Fig. 6-38 demonstrating benign spindle cells (hematoxylin–eosin, original magnification × 150). (Courtesy of Dr. John Finlay.)

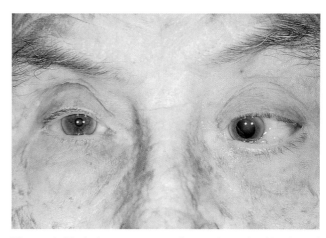

Figure 6-40. Leiomyosarcoma. Proptosis and adduction of the left eye in an 82-year-old woman.

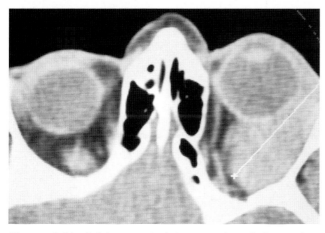

Figure 6-41. Axial computed tomography of the patient shown in Fig. 6-40 revealing a large mass in the retrobulbar space and temporal aspect of the orbit.

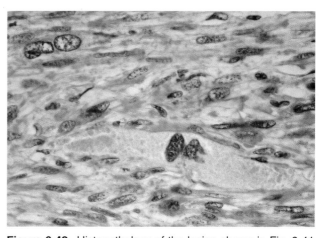

Figure 6-42. Histopathology of the lesion shown in Fig. 6-41 demonstrating malignant spindle cells. Electron microscopy confirmed the smooth muscle origin of the cells (hematoxylin–eosin, original magnification × 150).

CHAPTER 7

Fibrous Connective-Tissue Tumors

NODULAR FASCIITIS, FIBROMA, FIBROMATOSIS, AND FIBROSARCOMA

Mass lesions composed mainly of fibroblastic cells include nodular fasciitis, fibroma, fibromatosis, and fibrosarcoma. Each of these conditions may be very similar clinically and histopathologically. Nodular fasciitis is a benign nodular proliferation of connective tissue that usually involves the superficial fascia. It now is recognized to occur in the ocular adnexa and deeper in the orbit. Like other reactive inflammatory processes, it tends to have a rapid onset and progression. It has a tendency to occur in younger patients (1–4). Histopathologically, it is composed of well-defined sheets of primitive active fibroblasts, sometimes with acute and chronic inflammatory cells. Like other well-defined orbital masses, it usually is managed by surgical excision.

Fibroma is an idiopathic, benign, circumscribed tumor composed of well-differentiated fibroblasts (1,5). It sometimes can be diffuse or multinodular. It usually is not diagnosed clinically but rather in the pathology laboratory after excision, which is the treatment of choice.

The fibromatoses (myofibromatoses) are a group of nonencapsulated, nonmetastasizing fibrous tumors that involve orbital soft tissue and bone. They have a tendency toward local recurrence following surgical excision (1,6–8). It may occur at any age and may be confined to the orbit or a part of generalized fibromatoses. It can occur at a young age (juvenile fibromatosis) and may be diffuse, clinically resembling the plexiform neurofibroma of von Recklinghausen's disease. Histopathologically, it is composed of interlacing bundles of fibroblasts in a collagenous background matrix.

Fibrosarcoma is a proliferation of fibroblasts that exhibits malignant features clinically and histopathologically (9). It can occur as a primary tumor in children or adults, and it can occur after radiation therapy for familial retinoblastoma (1,8). The preferred management is wide surgical excision, including orbital exenteration if necessary. Supplemental irradiation and chemotherapy may be warranted.

SELECTED REFERENCES

1. Shields JA. *Diagnosis and management of orbital tumors.* Philadelphia: WB Saunders, 1989:192–204.
2. Font RL, Zimmerman LE. Nodular fasciitis of the eye and adnexa. A report of ten cases. *Arch Ophthalmol* 1966;75;475–481.
3. Levitt JM, deVeer A, Oguzhan C. Orbital nodular fasciitis. *Arch Ophthalmol* 1969;81:235—237.
4. Perry R, Ramani P, Mc Allister V, et al. Nodular fasciitis causing unilateral proptosis. *Br J Ophthalmol* 1975; 59:404–408.
5. Mortada AK. Fibroma of the orbit. *Br J Ophthalmol* 1971;55:350–352.
6. Hidayat AA, Font RL. Juvenile fibromatosis of the periorbital region and eyelid. A clinicopathologic study of six cases. *Arch Ophthalmol* 1980;98:280–285.
7. Waltermann JM, Huntrakoon M, Beatty EC Jr, Cibis GW. Congenital fibromatosis (myofibromatosis). A rare cause of proptosis at birth. *Ann Ophthalmol* 1988;20:394–399.
8. Shields CL, Husson M, Shields JA, Mercado G, Eagle RC Jr. Solitary intraosseous infantile myofibroma of the orbital roof. *Arch Ophthalmol* 1998;116:1528–1530.
9. Weiner JM, Hidayat AA. Juvenile fibrosarcoma of the orbit and eyelid. A study of five cases. *Arch Ophthalmol* 1983;101:253–259.

Nodular Fasciitis and Fibroma

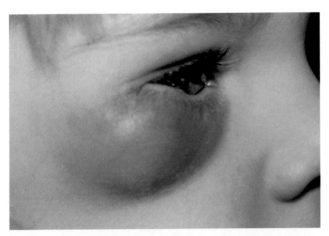

Figure 7-1. Nodular fasciitis in the inferior orbit and subcutaneous tissue in a 2-year-old girl. (Courtesy of Dr. Mark Ost.)

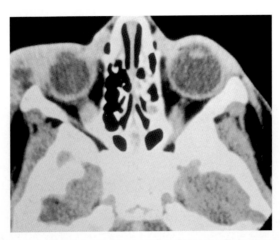

Figure 7-2. Axial computed tomography of the patient shown in Figure 7-1 demonstrating the tumor in the inferotemporal aspect of the orbit and subcutaneous tissue. (Courtesy of Dr. Mark Ost.)

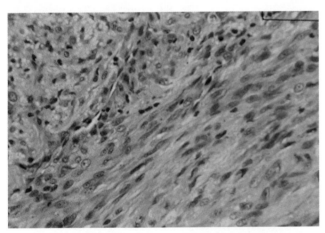

Figure 7-3. Histopathology of nodular fasciitis demonstrating sheets of proliferating fibroblasts and chronic inflammatory cells (hematoxylin–eosin, original magnification × 150).

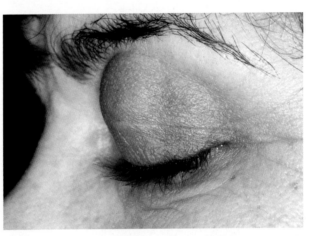

Figure 7-4. Fibroma of the superior orbit and subcutaneous tissue in a 49-year-old woman. It had been noticed 1 year earlier and had not shown appreciable change. (Courtesy of Dr. Mourad Khalil.)

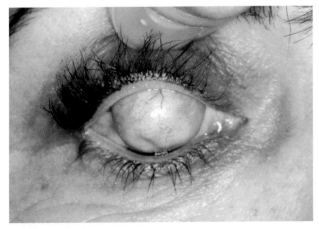

Figure 7-5. Same lesion shown in Fig. 7-4 with eyelid elevated. Note the smooth, circumscribed appearance of the lesion. (Courtesy of Dr. Mourad Khalil.)

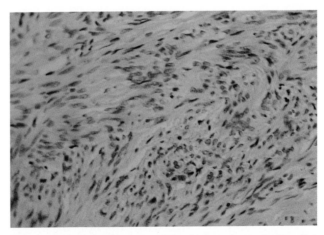

Figure 7-6. Histopathology of the lesion shown in Fig. 7-4 demonstrating closely packed fibrocytes consistent with fibroma (hematoxylin–eosin, original magnification × 150). (Courtesy of Dr. Mourad Khalil.)

Fibromatosis

Figs. 7-7 through 7-9 from Shields CL, Husson M, Shields JA, Eagle RC Jr. Solitary intraosseous infantile myofibroma of the orbital roof. *Arch Ophthalmol* 1998;116: 1528–1530.

Figs. 7-10 through 7-12 courtesy of Dr. Gerhard Cibis. From Waltermann JM, Huntrakoon M, Beatty EC Jr, Cibis GW. Congenital fibromatosis (myofibromatosis). A rare cause of proptosis at birth. *Ann Ophthalmol* 1988;20:394–399.

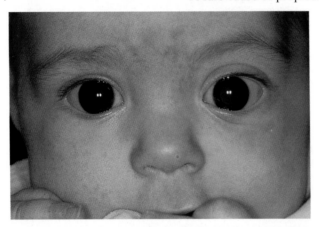

Figure 7-7. Infantile fibromatosis in a 1-month-old girl. Slight proptosis of the left eye was noted shortly after birth.

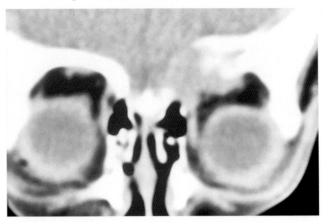

Figure 7-8. Coronal computed tomography of the child shown in Fig. 7-7 demonstrating a superonasal bone-destructive lesion involving the sphenoid bone.

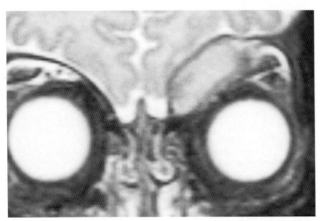

Figure 7-9. Coronal computed tomography in T2-weighted image with gadolinium enhancement showing the mildly enhancing superonasal mass.

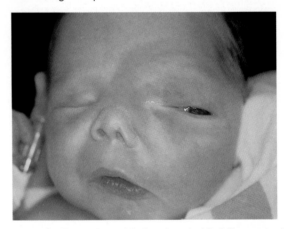

Figure 7-10. Extensive orbital and periorbital fibromatosis in a newborn boy.

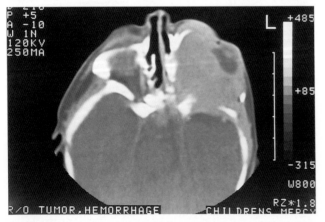

Figure 7-11. Axial computed tomography of the child shown in Fig. 7-10. The tumor filled the entire orbit and ethmoid and extended into the cranial cavity of other sections.

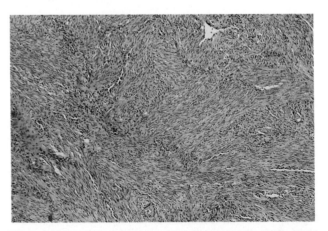

Figure 7-12. Histopathology of the lesion shown in Fig. 7-11 demonstrating benign spindle cells compatible with fibromatosis (hematoxylin–eosin, original magnification × 80).

Fibrosarcoma

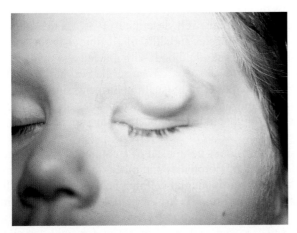

Figure 7-13. Localized fibrosarcoma of the superior orbit presenting as a subcutaneous mass in the eyebrow area in a 6-year-old girl.

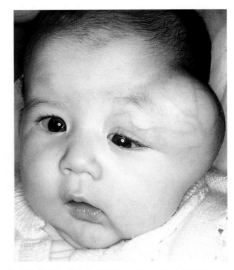

Figure 7-14. Massive orbital and periorbital fibrosarcoma in an infant. (Courtesy of Dr. Eduardo Arenas.)

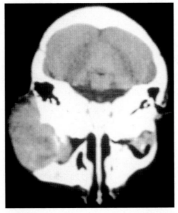

Figure 7-15. Axial computed tomography of the child shown in Fig. 7-14 demonstrating involvement of the orbital and temporal fossa by the large mass. (Courtesy of Dr. Eduardo Arenas.)

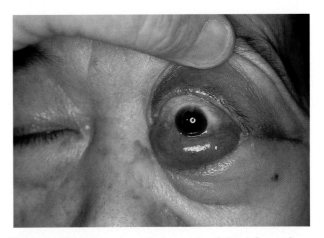

Figure 7-16. Proptosis and chemosis of the left eye in an elderly man, secondary to orbital fibrosarcoma. (Courtesy of Dr. Charles Lee.)

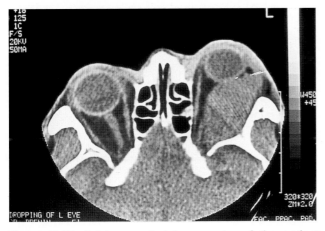

Figure 7-17. Axial computed tomography of the patient shown in Fig. 7-16 demonstrating the large orbital tumor. (Courtesy of Dr. Charles Lee.)

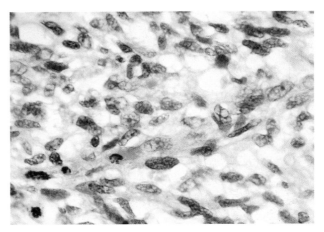

Figure 7-18. Histopathology of the lesion shown in Fig. 7-17 demonstrating malignant spindle cells. There was some debate as to the exact diagnosis, but most authorities favored the diagnosis of fibrosarcoma. (Courtesy of Dr. Charles Lee.)

FIBROUS HISTIOCYTOMA

Fibrous histiocytoma is perhaps the most common mesenchymal tumor of the orbit. The clinical and histopathologic features are well described (1–3). In the author's series, it accounted for 1% of all orbital biopsies and 80% of all fibrous tissue orbital tumors (4). It usually has its clinical onset in adulthood, with a mean age of 43 years at the time of diagnosis (2). It usually presents as a circumscribed orbital mass that produces proptosis, displacement of the globe, and visual impairment, similar to cavernous hemangioma, neurilemoma, and other circumscribed orbital masses. It can occur anywhere in the orbit, but has a slight tendency to occur in the superior and nasal extraconal areas.

Histopathologically, fibrous histiocytoma is composed of a combined proliferation of cells, some of which exhibit features of fibroblasts and others that exhibit features of histiocytes. It possibly arises from a pluripotential cell that has the capacity to differentiate into either fibroblasts or histiocytes. Based on pathologic criteria, orbital fibrous histiocytoma has been divided into benign (63%), locally aggressive (26%), and malignant categories (11%) (2). Frozen sections with stains for lipid can show positive reaction in the histiocytes, supporting the diagnosis. Management is complete surgical resection of the mass within its capsule. Incomplete excision can lead to recurrence and possible malignant transformation.

SELECTED REFERENCES

1. Shields JA. *Diagnosis and management of orbital tumors.* Philadelphia: WB Saunders, 1989:192–204.
2. Font RL, Hidayat AA. Fibrous histiocytoma of the orbit. *Hum Pathol* 1982;13:199–209.
3. Jakobiec FA, Howard GM, Gones IS, et al. Fibrous histiocytoma of the orbit. *Am J Ophthalmol* 1974;77:333–345.
4. Shields JA, Bakewell B, Augsburger JJ, Flanagan JC. Classification and incidence of space-occupying lesions of the orbit. A survey of 645 biopsies. *Arch Ophthalmol* 1984;102:1606–1611.

Benign Fibrous Histiocytoma

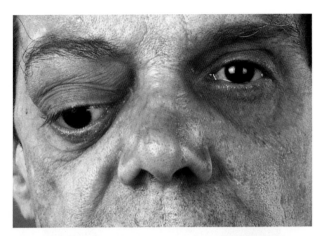

Figure 7-19. Benign fibrous histiocytoma. Proptosis and downward displacement of the left eye in a 49-year-old man. (Courtesy of Dr. Norman Charles.)

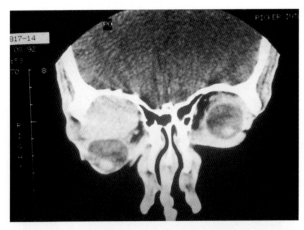

Figure 7-20. Coronal computed tomography of the patient shown in Fig. 7-19 showing well-circumscribed superior orbital mass. (Courtesy of Dr. Norman Charles.)

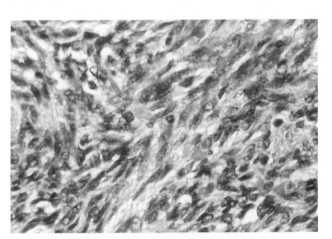

Figure 7-21. Histopathology of the lesion shown in Fig. 7-20. There are fascicles of spindle cells with interspersed histiocytes (hematoxylin–eosin, original magnification × 200). (Courtesy of Dr. Norman Charles.)

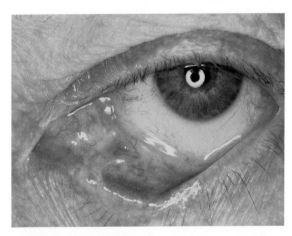

Figure 7-22. Conjunctival mass and ectropion of the right lower eyelid in a 62-year-old man. (Courtesy of Dr. Douglas Cameron.)

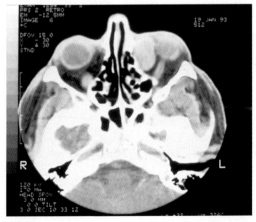

Figure 7-23. Axial computed tomography of the patient shown in Fig. 7-22 depicting a characteristic, well-circumscribed nasal orbital mass. (Courtesy of Dr. Douglas Cameron.)

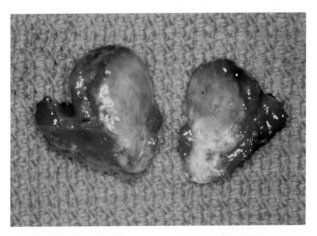

Figure 7-24. Gross appearance of the sectioned lesion after surgical excision. Note the yellow appearance of the mass, a feature that is characteristic of fibrous histiocytoma. (Courtesy of Dr. Douglas Cameron.)

Malignant Fibrous Histiocytoma

Locally invasive histiocytoma and malignant fibrous histiocytoma are grouped together because both can exhibit malignant behavior. The former tends to grow locally and the latter has the additional capacity to metastasize. The benign, locally aggressive, and malignant types usually are impossible to differentiate clinically, and the diagnosis and classification is made on histopathologic examination.

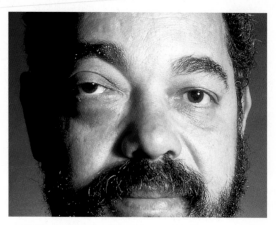

Figure 7-25. Locally invasive fibrous histiocytoma. Proptosis and lateral displacement of the right eye in a 42-year-old man. (Courtesy of Dr. Norman Charles.)

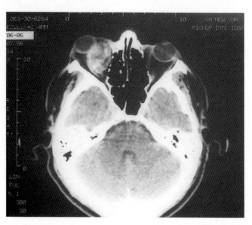

Figure 7-26. Axial computed tomography of the patient shown in Fig. 7-25 demonstrating the circumscribed nasal orbital mass. The lesion was excised and classified as a locally invasive fibrous histiocytoma. (Courtesy of Dr. Norman Charles.)

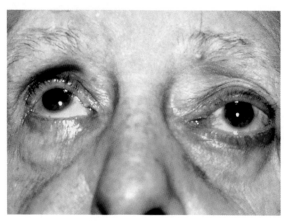

Figure 7-27. Malignant fibrous histiocytoma. Proptosis and restriction of upgaze in left eye of an 85-year-old woman. (Courtesy of Dr. Martha Farber.)

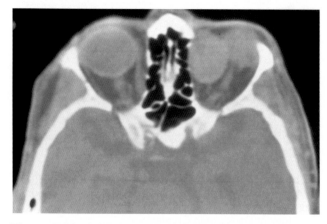

Figure 7-28. Axial computed tomography of the patient shown in Fig. 7-27 revealing ovoid, circumscribed nasal orbital mass. (Courtesy of Dr. Martha Farber.)

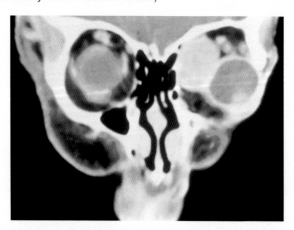

Figure 7-29. Coronal computed tomography of the lesion shown in Fig. 7-28 depicting the shape and location of the superonasal orbital mass. (Courtesy of Dr. Martha Farber.)

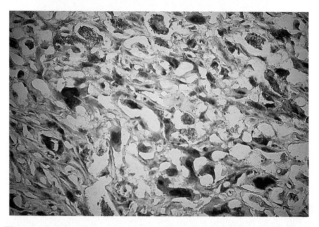

Figure 7-30. Histopathology of malignant fibrous histiocytoma showing pleomorphic cells and positive staining for lipid (oil red-O, original magnification × 200). (Courtesy of Armed Forces Institute of Pathology, Washington, DC.)

Fibrous Histiocytoma—Management

The goal of treatment is complete excision of the mass within its capsule or pseudo-capsule in order to prevent recurrence and malignant transformation. A case example of a patient referred for excision of a recurrent benign fibrous histiocytoma is shown.

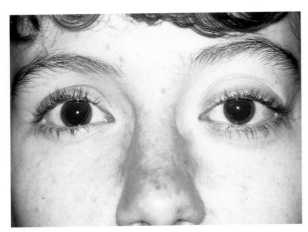

Figure 7-31. Proptosis of the left eye secondary to orbital fibrous histiocytoma in a 24-year-old woman.

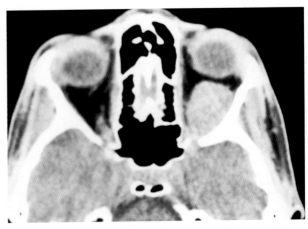

Figure 7-32. Axial computed tomography showing circumscribed orbital mass.

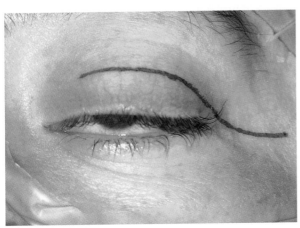

Figure 7-33. Planned superotemporal eyelid crease incision to remove the tumor.

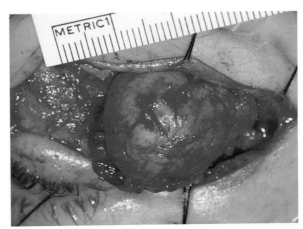

Figure 7-34. Tumor exposed at the time of superolateral orbitotomy.

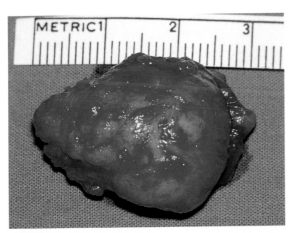

Figure 7-35. Gross appearance of the lesion, which is about 30 mm in its largest diameter.

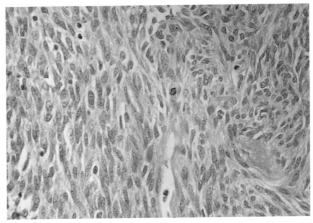

Figure 7-36. Histopathology of fibrous histiocytoma (hematoxylin–eosin, original magnification × 150).

CHAPTER 8

Osseous, Fibroosseous, and Cartilaginous Tumors

OSTEOMA

The orbital bones can give rise to benign tumors (osteoma) or malignant neoplasms (osteosarcoma) (1,2). Most osteomas in the orbital region arise from the bones in the paranasal sinuses and do not produce orbital signs (1). Some, however, originate in the orbital bones and protrude mainly into the orbit. Depending on the location of the osteoma, there may be displacement of the globe and proptosis. Orbital osteoma sometimes can occur with Gardner's syndrome, a familial condition characterized by adenomatous polyposis of the bowel, secondary bowel cancer, typical congenital hyperplastic lesions of the retinal pigment epithelium, and other findings (3,4). Computed tomography of orbital osteoma shows a round or lobular mass of bone density arising from otherwise normal bone. The ivory type may be identical to bone. The fibrous type is less dense and may resemble fibrous dysplasia.

Histopathologically, the ivory variant is mostly bony trabeculae with little fibrous tissue. The mature type has thinner trabeculae and more fibrous tissue. The fibrous type has more extensive fibrous tissue and can resemble fibrous dysplasia of bone (1,2). Management is observation of the small asymptomatic lesions and excision, using bone instruments, of the larger or symptomatic ones.

SELECTED REFERENCES

1. Shields JA. *Diagnosis and management of orbital tumors.* Philadelphia: WB Saunders, 1989:205–211.
2. Grove AS. Osteomas of the orbit. *Ophthalmic Surg* 1978;9:23–39.
3. Whitson WE, Orcutt JC, Walkinshaw MD. Orbital osteoma in Gardner's syndrome. *Am J Ophthalmol* 1986; 101:236–241.
4. Van Gehuchten D, Lemagne JM, Weber S, Michiels J. A case of exophthalmos—an early symptom of Gardner's syndrome. *Orbit* 1982;1:61–69.

Osteoma

Figs. 8-5 and 8-6 courtesy of Dr. James Orcutt. From Whitson WE, Orcutt JC, Walkinshaw MD. Orbital osteoma in Gardner's syndrome. *Am J Ophthalmol* 1986;101:236–241.

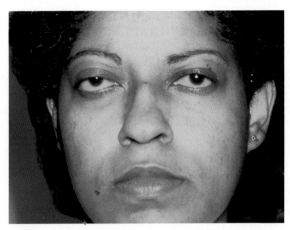

Figure 8-1. Orbital osteoma. Proptosis of the right eye in a 26-year-old woman. (Courtesy of Drs. Pearl Rosenbaum and Thomas Slamovitz.)

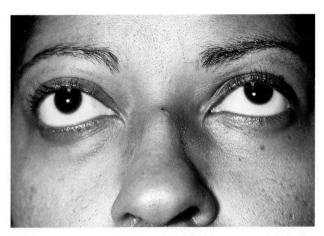

Figure 8-2. Patient shown in Fig. 8-1 demonstrating limitation of supraduction of the right eye.

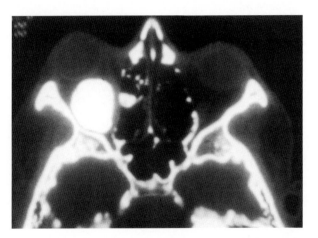

Figure 8-3. Axial computed tomography of the patient shown in Fig. 8-1 demonstrating a dense mass involving the orbital roof and part of the ethmoid sinus.

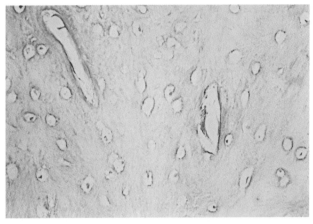

Figure 8-4. Histopathology of the lesion shown in Fig. 8-3 demonstrating compact bone and minimal fibrous stroma (hematoxylin–eosin, original magnification × 50).

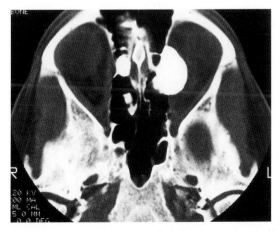

Figure 8-5. Orbital osteoma in Gardner's syndrome. Axial computed tomography showing large bone density mass originating from the medial orbital wall.

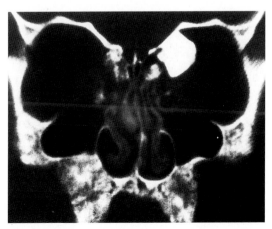

Figure 8-6. Coronal computed tomography of the lesion shown in Fig. 8-5.

OSTEOSARCOMA

Osteosarcoma (osteogenic sarcoma) is a highly malignant tumor that can affect the orbital bones as a primary lesion or as a secondary tumor after irradiation for familial retinoblastoma (1–4). It can occur at any age and can arise from any of the orbital bones, producing a variety of orbital signs and symptoms. It is generally a progressive lesion that can produce proptosis, displacement of the globe, pain, periorbital numbness, eyelid edema, and conjunctival chemosis. Computed tomography shows a destructive lesion of affected bone. Histopathologically, osteosarcoma consists of anaplastic malignant spindle cells with osteoid and neoplastic bone formation. Most arise *de novo*, but osteosarcoma occasionally can occur from chronic bone diseases such as Paget's disease and fibrous dysplasia (3). The management is wide surgical resection often combined with irradiation and chemotherapy. The prognosis is guarded.

SELECTED REFERENCES

1. Shields JA. *Diagnosis and management of orbital tumors.* Philadelphia: WB Saunders, 1989:205–211.
2. Dhir SP, Munjal VP, Jain IS, et al. Osteosarcoma of the orbit. *J Pediatr Ophthalmol Strabismus* 1980;17: 312–314.
3. Blodi FC. Pathology of orbital bones. The XXXII Edward Jackson Memorial Lecture. *Am J Ophthalmol* 1976;81:1–26.
4. Abramson DH, Ronner HJ, Ellsworth RM. Second tumors in irradiated bilateral retinoblastoma. *Am J Ophthalmol* 1979;87:624–628.

Osteosarcoma

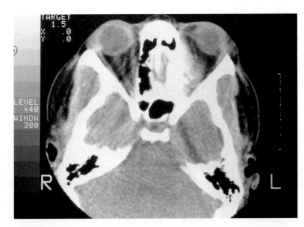

Figure 8-7. Axial computed tomography of a 19-year-old woman with no prior history of retinoblastoma who presented with proptosis of the left eye. Note the diffuse mass in the medial aspect of the orbit with involvement of the ethmoid sinus. (Courtesy of Dr. Elise Torczynski.)

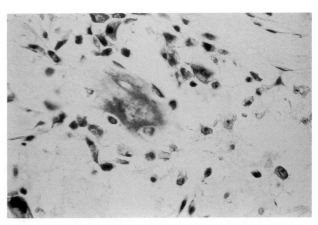

Figure 8-8. Histopathology of the lesion shown in Fig. 8-7 showing neoplastic cells in a myxomatous matrix (hematoxylin–eosin, original magnification × 200). (Courtesy of Dr. Elise Torczynski.)

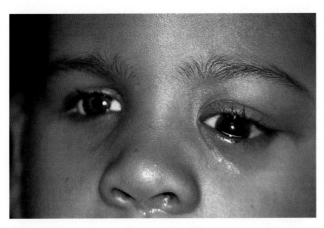

Figure 8-9. Facial appearance of a 5-year-old child who at age 1 year had undergone enucleation of the right eye and irradiation of the left eye for retinoblastoma.

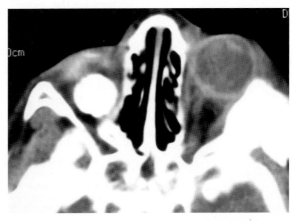

Figure 8-10. Axial computed tomography of the child shown in Fig. 8-9. Note the orbital implant on the right side and the extensive bony mass superotemporally in the orbit on the left side.

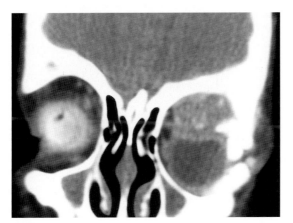

Figure 8-11. Coronal computed tomography of the child shown in Fig. 8-9. Note the soft-tissue component in the superior portion of the left orbit.

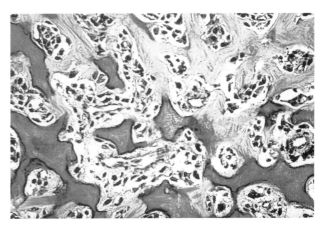

Figure 8-12. Histopathology of another case of osteosarcoma (hematoxylin–eosin, original magnification × 100). (Courtesy of Armed Forces Institute of Pathology, Washington, DC.)

FIBROUS DYSPLASIA

There are several closely related fibroosseous lesions that can occur in the orbital bones, including fibrous dysplasia, ossifying fibroma, aneurysmal bone cyst, giant-cell tumor (osteoclastoma), giant-cell reparative granuloma, and brown tumor of hyperparathyroidism. Most of these are discussed in more detail elsewhere (1), but some are discussed and illustrated here.

Fibrous dysplasia is a fibroosseous lesion that is considered to be a hamartomatous malformation resulting from an idiopathic arrest of the maturation of bone at the woven bone stage. It generally has its onset in the first or second decade (1,2). Because the frontal bone is most often involved, there is usually proptosis and downward displacement of the globe. Less often, it can occur in the ethmoid or maxillary bones. Fibrous dysplasia can be monostotic or polyostotic, the latter being sometimes associated with Albright's syndrome, characterized by precocious puberty in females and mottled skin pigmentation ipsilateral to the osseous involvement (3). Most orbital cases are not associated with Albright's syndrome.

Histopathologically, fibrous dysplasia is composed of benign spindle cells in a fibrous tissue stroma and trabeculae of immature woven bone without osteoblasts. This feature helps differentiate fibrous dysplasia from ossifying fibroma, which does have osteoblasts.

Management of fibrous dysplasia of the orbital bones generally is observation, because the lesion may be relatively stable for many years. Visual acuity, pupillary evaluation, color vision, visual fields, and coronal computed tomographic studies of the optic canals should be done periodically. If the process encroaches on the optic canal or becomes cosmetically unacceptable, then surgical resection should be undertaken, usually in conjunction with a neurosurgeon or otolaryngologist, combined with craniofacial reconstruction. Fibrous dysplasia has been known to undergo malignant transformation into osteosarcoma, fibrosarcoma, and other tumors (4).

SELECTED REFERENCES

1. Shields JA. *Diagnosis and management of orbital tumors.* Philadelphia: WB Saunders, 1989:219–221.
2. Moore RT. Fibrous dysplasia of the orbit. *Rev Surv Ophthalmol* 1969;13:321–334.
3. Moore AT, Buncic JR, Munro IR. Fibrous dysplasia of the orbit in childhood. Clinical features and management. *Ophthalmology* 1985;92:12–20.
4. Liakos GM, Walder CB, Carruth JAS. Ocular complications in craniofacial fibrous dysplasia. *Br J Ophthalmol* 1979;63:611–66.

Fibrous Dysplasia

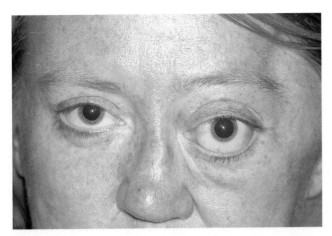

Figure 8-13. Left proptosis and swelling of the temporal fossa in a 38-year-old woman with fibrous dysplasia.

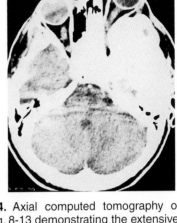

Figure 8-14. Axial computed tomography of the patient shown in Fig. 8-13 demonstrating the extensive mass involving the orbit, temporal fossa, and cranial cavity.

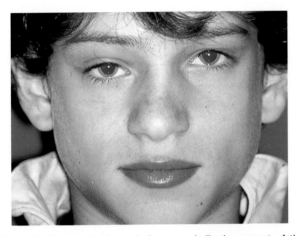

Figure 8-15. Proptosis and downward displacement of the right eye in a 13-year-old boy with fibrous dysplasia.

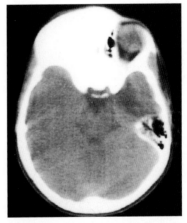

Figure 8-16. Axial computed tomography through the superior aspect of the orbit of the patient shown in Fig. 8-15 demonstrating the extent of the bony lesion.

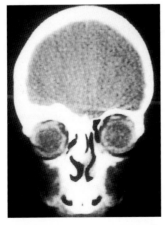

Figure 8-17. Coronal computed tomography of the patient shown in Fig. 8-15 demonstrating diffuse thickening of the frontal bone.

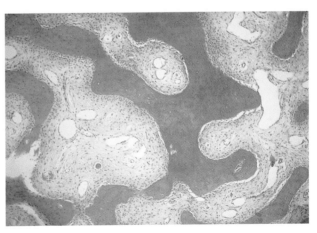

Figure 8-18. Histopathology of fibrous dysplasia showing immature woven bone (hematoxylin–eosin, original magnification × 50).

OSSIFYING FIBROMA

Ossifying fibroma is an acquired benign tumor of bone, in contrast to fibrous dysplasia, which is believed to an arrest in the normal development of bone (1–4). Ossifying fibroma has its clinical onset early in life (mean age 15 years) and therefore is called juvenile ossifying fibroma (1–4). There is gradual proptosis and displacement of the globe, the direction depending on which orbital bones are affected. Involvement of the adjacent sinuses is the rule. Clinically, ossifying fibroma seems to be more aggressive than fibrous dysplasia. Computed tomography demonstrates a localized expansion of the involved bone, which may appear homogeneously opaque on standard settings and more heterogeneous with bone window settings.

On low-magnification histopathology, ossifying fibroma appears like a spindle cell tumor, with bony foci that closely resemble psammoma bodies that characterize meningioma. Such lesions occasionally are misdiagnosed as meningioma. Hence, the tumor has been called psammomatoid ossifying fibroma (2). On higher power, however, the focal areas are irregular bony foci and appear different from psammoma bodies.

Management of orbital ossifying fibroma is surgical removal. Most affected patients have developed progressive symptoms that make early surgical removal justified in most cases, combined with craniofacial reconstruction (1–4).

SELECTED REFERENCES

1. Shields JA. *Diagnosis and management of orbital tumors.* Philadelphia: WB Saunders, 1989:221–222.
2. Margo CE, Ragsdale BD, Perman KI, Zimmerman LE, Sweet DE. Psammomatoid (juvenile) ossifying fibroma of the orbit. *Ophthalmology* 1985;92;150–159.
3. Shields JA, Nelson LB, Brown JF, Dolinskas C. Clinical, computed tomographic, and histopathologic characteristics of juvenile ossifying fibroma with orbital involvement. *Am J Ophthalmol* 1983;96:650–653.
4. Shields JA, Peyster RG, Augsburger JJ, Kapustiak J, Handler SD. Massive juvenile ossifying fibroma of maxillary sinus with orbital involvement. *Br J Ophthalmol* 1985;69:392–395.

Ossifying Fibroma

Figs. 8-21 through 8-23 from Shields JA, Peyster RG, Augsburger JJ, Kapustiak J, Handler SD. Massive juvenile ossifying fibroma of maxillary sinus with orbital involvement. *Br J Ophthalmol* 1985;69:392–395.

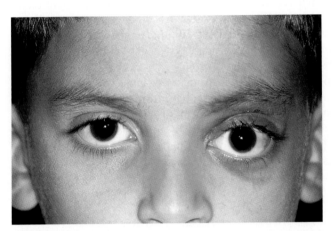

Figure 8-19. Proptosis and downward displacement of the left eye in an 8-year-old boy.

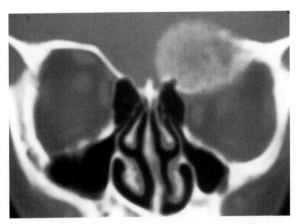

Figure 8-20. Coronal computed tomography of the patient shown in Fig. 8-19 demonstrating the ovoid heterogeneous mass of the frontal bone and the orbital roof.

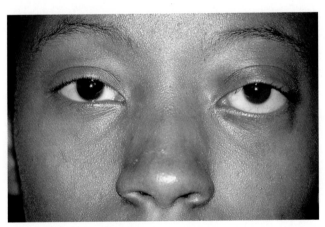

Figure 8-21. Proptosis and upward displacement of the left eye in a 14-year-old girl.

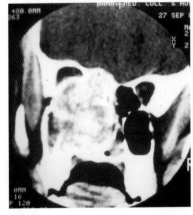

Figure 8-22. Coronal computed tomography of the patient shown in Fig. 8-21 demonstrating the large mass in the maxillary sinus invading through the floor of the orbit.

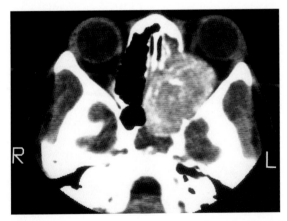

Figure 8-23. Axial computed tomography of the patient shown in Fig. 8-21 demonstrating involvement of the posterior aspect of the orbit by the lesion.

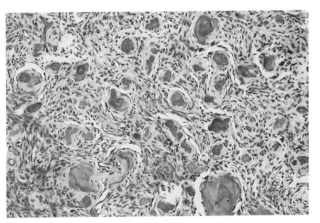

Figure 8-24. Histopathology showing fibrous tissue and ossicles that resemble psammoma bodies (hematoxylin–eosin, original magnification × 100).

GIANT-CELL REPARATIVE GRANULOMA

Giant-cell reparative granuloma is a benign fibroosseous lesion that usually occurs in the mandible. It occasionally can involve the bones of the skull and orbit (1–3). In the orbit, it generally occurs in children and young adults as a slowly progressive lesion in the orbital roof, which can cause proptosis, downward displacement of the globe, diplopia, pain, and visual loss. With imaging studies, it appears as a fibroosseous mass with features similar to ossifying fibroma or aneurysmal bone cyst, often with blood cysts. Clinically and radiographically, it may closely resemble an organizing subperiosteal abscess in the superior orbit.

Histopathologically, it consists of a fibrous stroma with giant cells, spindle cells, and organizing blood. It may be difficult to differentiate from organizing hematoma, giant-cell tumor, brown tumor or hyperparathyroidism, or other fibroosseous lesions.

The usual management is surgical excision, usually by curettage. Supplemental systemic corticosteroids may hasten resolution of residual mass. Radiotherapy can be attempted for difficult cases, but generally it is not advisable.

SELECTED REFERENCES

1. Shields JA. *Diagnosis and management of orbital tumors.* Philadelphia: WB Saunders, 1989:217–219.
2. Hoopes PC, Anderson RI, Blodi FC. Giant cell (reparative) granuloma of the orbit. *Ophthalmology* 1981;88: 1361–1366.
3. Mercado GV, Shields CL, Gunduz K, Shields JA, Eagle RC Jr. Giant cell reparative granuloma of the orbit *Am J Ophthalmol (in press).*

Giant-cell Reparative Granuloma

A clinicopathologic correlation of a lesion diagnosed as a giant-cell granuloma is shown. The initial diagnosis was aneurysmal bone cysts, but most ophthalmic pathology consultations favored the diagnosis of giant-cell reparative granuloma.

From Mercado GV, Shields CL, Gunduz K, Shields JA, Eagle RC Jr. Giant cell reparative granuloma of the orbit. *Am J Ophthalmol (in press)*.

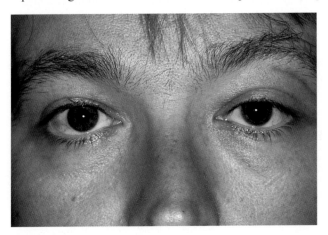

Figure 8-25. Proptosis of the left eye in a 38-year-old man. Patient is shown after an incisional biopsy was done.

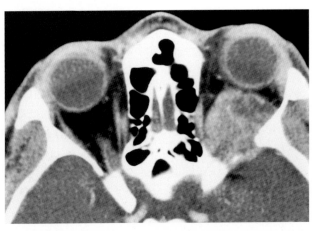

Figure 8-26. Axial computed tomography showing fairly well-defined mass near the orbital apex. Note the involvement of the lateral wall of the orbit.

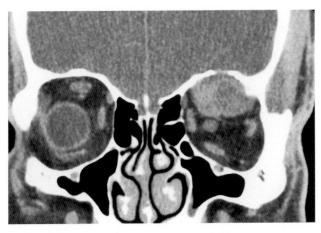

Figure 8-27. Coronal computed tomography showing the same mass in the orbit superiorly with involvement of the bone roof of the orbit.

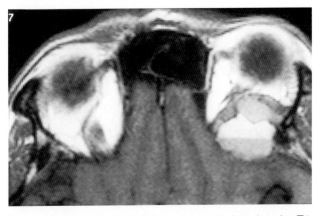

Figure 8-28. Axial magnetic resonance imaging in T1-weighted image demonstrating the cystic character of the lesion with a blood layer.

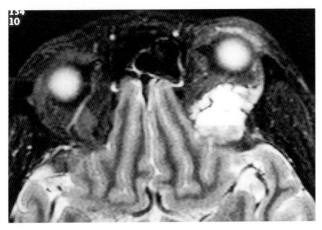

Figure 8-29. Axial magnetic resonance imaging through adjacent area with T2-weighted image further depicting the blood layer in the lesion.

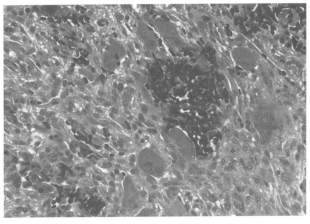

Figure 8-30. Histopathology showing dense fibrous tissue, blood, and giant cells (hematoxylin–eosin, original magnification × 150).

CHONDROMA

Cartilaginous tumors of the orbit can be benign (chondroma) or malignant (chondrosarcoma) (1–3). The trochlea of the superior oblique muscle is the only cartilaginous tissue in the orbit. A mass that arises from the mature cartilaginous trochlea is designated a true chondroma. A tumor that develops from primitive mesenchyma destined to form mature cartilage is better designated as cartilaginous hamartoma. True chondroma is exceedingly rare, and cartilaginous hamartoma occasionally is recognized in the orbit. Histopathologically, chondroma and cartilaginous hamartoma are composed of lobules of well-differentiated cartilage. Management is complete excision if possible.

SELECTED REFERENCES

1. Shields JA. *Diagnosis and management of orbital tumors.* Philadelphia: WB Saunders, 1989:223–225.
2. Bowen JH, Christensen FH, Klintworth GK, Syndor CF. A clinicopathologic study of a cartilaginous hamartoma of the orbit. A rare cause of proptosis. *Ophthalmology* 1981;88:1356–1360.
3. Jepson CN, Wetzig PC. Pure chondroma of the trochlea. *Surv Ophthalmol* 1966;11:656–659.

Chondroma

Figs. 8-31 through 8-34 courtesy of Dr. Gordon Klintworth. From Bowen JH, Christensen FH, Klintworth GK, Syndor CF. A clinicopathologic study of a cartilaginous hamartoma of the orbit. A rare cause of proptosis. *Ophthalmology* 1981;88:1356–1360.

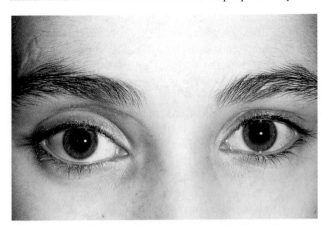

Figure 8-31. Cartilaginous hamartoma of the orbit. Proptosis of the right eye in an 11-year-old girl. The proptosis had been present for about 6 years. Computed tomography disclosed a circumscribed mass in the superonasal aspect of the orbit.

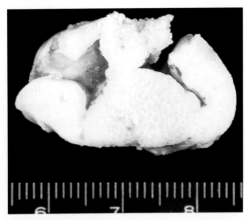

Figure 8-32. Gross appearance of the excised lesion from the patient shown in Fig. 8-31 showing multinodular pearly-white mass.

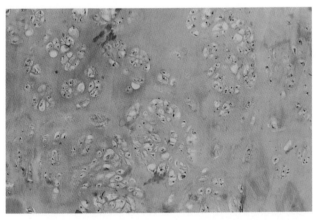

Figure 8-33. Histopathology of the lesion shown in Fig. 8-32 demonstrating mature cartilage (hematoxylin–eosin, original magnification × 100).

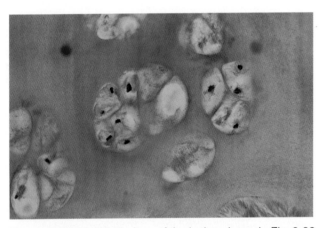

Figure 8-34. Histopathology of the lesion shown in Fig. 8-32 demonstrating mature cartilage (hematoxylin–eosin, original magnification × 200).

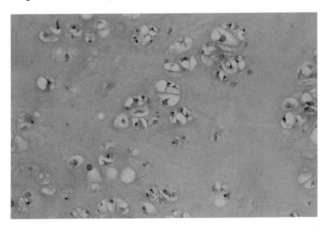

Figure 8-35. Acquired chondroma of the orbit. A 50-year-old man presented with a progressive hard mass in the superonasal aspect of the orbit. A mass corresponding to the location of the trochlea was excised. Photomicrograph depicts mature cartilage (hematoxylin–eosin, original magnification × 100). (Courtesy of Dr. Paul Wetzig.)

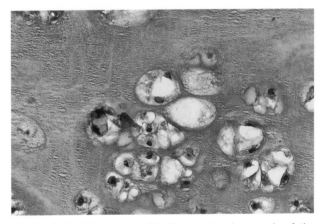

Figure 8-36. Higher-magnification photomicrograph of the lesion shown in Fig. 8-35 (hematoxylin–eosin, original magnification × 200). (Courtesy of Dr. Paul Wetzig.)

CHONDROSARCOMA

Chondrosarcoma is a malignant neoplasm of bone that is composed mainly of anaplastic chondrocytes. It most often occurs in the long bones but can develop in ribs, shoulder, pelvis, and occasionally in the orbital region. It usually originates in the bones of the nasal cavity or sinuses and secondarily involves the orbit. It also can develop following radiotherapy for the germinal form of retinoblastoma (1). Low-grade orbital chondrosarcoma also is known to arise in periorbital areas of involvement by multiple enchondromatosis (Ollier's disease) (2).

The most common variant of chondrosarcoma in the orbit is mesenchymal chondrosarcoma (1,3,4). This tumor can arise from bone or from extraskeletal soft tissue, where it probably develops from primitive mesenchymal tissue that exhibits cartilaginous differentiation. It generally occurs in adults and produces proptosis and displacement of the globe, like other orbital tumors. Imaging studies show an irregular mass with densities corresponding to areas of cartilage and bone.

Histopathologically, mesenchymal chondrosarcoma is composed of rather poorly differentiated mesenchymal tissue with islands of well-differentiated cartilage. The best management of orbital chondrosarcoma is complete surgical excision. More advanced cases often require orbital exenteration to completely eradicate the tumor. Supplemental irradiation and chemotherapy may be attempted in advanced cases (3,4).

SELECTED REFERENCES

1. Shields JA. *Diagnosis and management of orbital tumors.* Philadelphia: WB Saunders, 1989:225–227.
2. De Laey JJ, De Schryver A, Kluyskens P, Kunnen M. Orbital involvement in Ollier's disease (multiple enchondromatosis). *Int Ophthalmol* 1982;5:149–154.
3. Guccion JG, Font RL, Enzinger FM, Zimmerman LE. Extraskeletal mesenchymal chondrosarcoma. *Arch Pathol* 1973;95:336–340.
4. Jacobs JL, Merriam JC, Chadburn A, Garvin J, Housepian E, Hilal SK. Mesenchymal chondrosarcoma of the orbit. Report of three new cases and review of the literature. *Cancer* 1994;73:399–405.

Chondrosarcoma

Figs. 8-41 and 8-42 courtesy of Dr. JJ De Laey. From De Laey JJ, De Schryver A, Kluyskens P, Kunnen M. Orbital involvement in Ollier's disease (multiple enchondromatosis). *Int Ophthalmol* 1982;5:149–154.

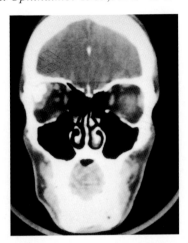

Figure 8-37. Coronal computed tomography of a 21-year-old man with superotemporal orbital mass. Note the bone and soft-tissue component of the mass.

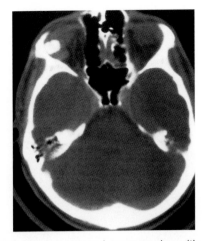

Figure 8-38. Axial computed tomography with bone windows of the lesion shown in Fig. 8-37 better depicting the bone density in the mass.

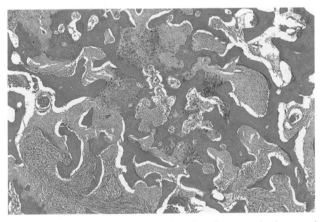

Figure 8-39. Histopathology showing bone spicules and connective tissue. Other areas showed more definitive cartilage (hematoxylin–eosin, original magnification × 80).

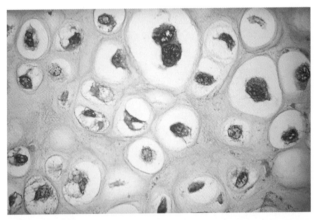

Figure 8-40. Photomicrograph of orbital chondrosarcoma from a child who had undergone irradiation for familial retinoblastoma, showing malignant chondroblasts (hematoxylin–eosin, original magnification × 250). (Courtesy of Armed Forces Institute of Pathology, Washington, DC.)

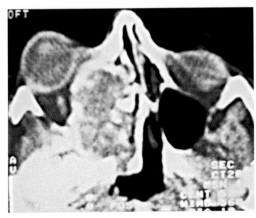

Figure 8-41. Chondrosarcoma associated with Ollier's disease. Axial computed tomography of a 52-year-old woman with Ollier's disease showing mass involving the nose and nasal aspect of the orbit.

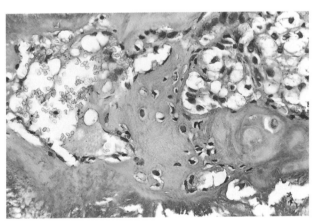

Figure 8-42. Histopathology of the lesion shown in Fig. 8-41 demonstrating well-differentiated chondrosarcoma (hematoxylin–eosin, original magnification × 75).

CHAPTER 9

Lipomatous and Myxomatous Tumors

HERNIATED ORBITAL FAT

Herniated (prolapsed) orbital fat is a spontaneous protrusion of orbital fat through a defect in Tenon's capsule. It differs from dermolipoma in that it occurs in older patients, is more often bilateral, is more elevated, and has readily visible lipid globules on slit-lamp examination. It is more compressible and becomes more prominent when the globe is gently pushed posteriorly, and it does not contain hairs (1).

Histopathologically, herniated orbital fat is composed of normal orbital fat. It can be managed by observation of surgical excision if the lesion is cosmetically unacceptable or producing symptoms of ocular irritation or dryness. The herniated anterior component can be excised by performing a conjunctival incision, clamping the posterior aspect of the lesion, and removing the fat with cutting cautery (1,2).

SELECTED REFERENCES

1. Jordan DR, Tse DT. Herniated orbital fat. *Can J Ophthalmol* 1987;22:173–177.
2. Schwartz F, Randall P. Conjunctival incision for herniated orbital fat. In: Wesley RE, ed. *Techniques in ophthalmic plastic surgery.* New York: John Wiley and Sons, 1996:55–58.

Herniated Orbital Fat

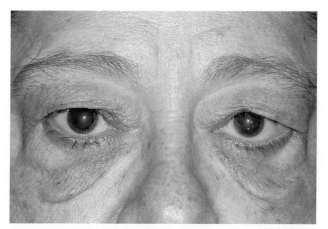

Figure 9-1. Bilateral herniated orbital fat producing bulging of the lower and upper eyelids in a 72-year-old woman.

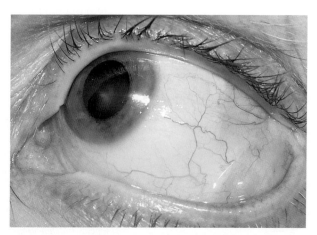

Figure 9-2. Inferotemporal herniated orbital fat in a 71-year-old woman.

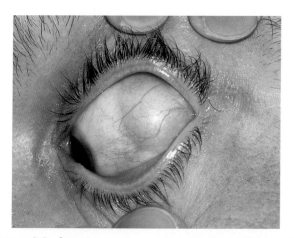

Figure 9-3. Superotemporal herniated orbital fat in a 51-year-old man. The lesion was progressive and excision was performed.

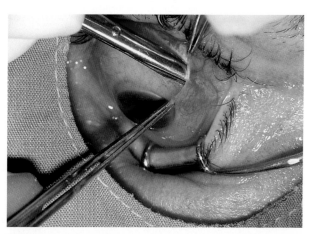

Figure 9-4. Forniceal conjunctival excision over the lesion to expose the mass for partial excision.

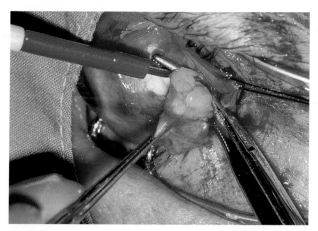

Figure 9-5. The fat has been exposed and clamped and is being cut.

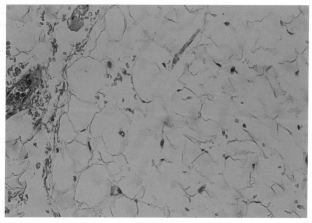

Figure 9-6. Histopathology of herniated orbital fat showing normal lipocytes.

DERMOLIPOMA

Dermolipoma is a benign congenital lesion that may be evident at birth or detected later in life (1). It usually is located in the anterior aspect of the orbit and may contain visible hairs. Its differentiation from herniated orbital fat is discussed in the prior section (2). Dermolipoma, like the limbal dermoid tumor, is often a part of Goldenhar's syndrome, in which instances it may be bilateral. It also can be a component of the epibulbar complex choristoma seen with the organoid nevus syndrome (3).

Histopathologically, dermolipoma is lined by stratified epithelium that may contain hair and have slight keratinization. The superficial subepithelial tissue is composed of dense collagen bundles and the deeper tissue contains mature fat (1). Smaller asymptomatic dermolipoma can be followed without treatment, and large symptomatic ones are managed by local excision. The prognosis is good.

SELECTED REFERENCES

1. Shields JA. *Diagnosis and management of orbital tumors.* Philadelphia: WB Saunders, 1989:236–238.
2. Jordan DR, Tse DT. Herniated orbital fat. *Can J Ophthalmol* 1987;22:173–177.
3. Shields JA, Shields CL, Eagle RC Jr, Arevalo F, De Potter P. Ocular manifestations of the organoid nevus syndrome. *Ophthalmology* 1997;104:549–557.

Dermolipoma

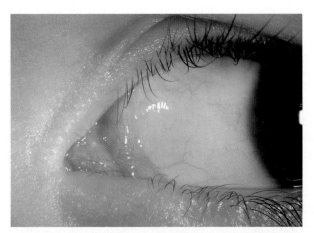

Figure 9-7. Dermolipoma presenting in the medial canthal region of a 2-year-old child with Goldenhar's syndrome.

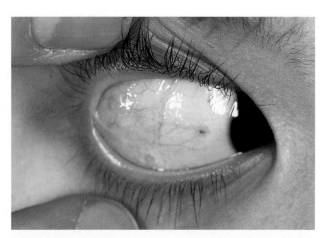

Figure 9-8. Dermolipoma presenting as a superotemporal orbitoconjunctival mass in a 6-year-old girl who had no evidence of Goldenhar's syndrome. (Courtesy of Dr. Norman Charles.)

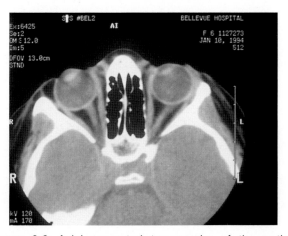

Figure 9-9. Axial computed tomography of the patient shown in Fig. 9-8 demonstrating a triangular lesion temporal to the right eye that has density identical to orbital fat. (Courtesy of Dr. Norman Charles.)

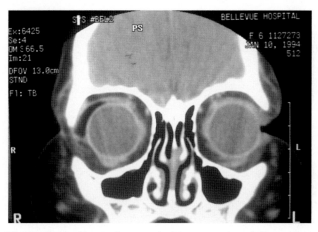

Figure 9-10. Coronal computed tomography of the patient shown in Fig. 9-8 depicting the same lesion superotemporal to the globe. (Courtesy of Dr. Norman Charles.)

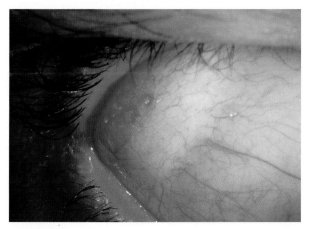

Figure 9-11. Orbitoconjunctival dermolipoma presenting in the superotemporal fornix of a 19-year-old man.

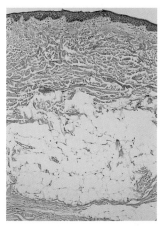

Figure 9-12. Histopathology of orbitoconjunctival dermolipoma showing epithelium, collagenous tissue, and deeper fat.

LIPOMA

Lipoma is a benign tumor composed of adipose tissue. It is relatively common in subcutaneous tissue in many parts of the body but is rare in the orbit (1). It is likely that some cases diagnosed as orbital lipoma actually may represent herniated orbital fat. Variations of lipoma, such as spindle cell lipoma (2,3), angiolipoma (4), and pleomorphic lipoma, have been recognized in the orbit. Myxoma, a closely related tumor, has been discussed elsewhere (5). Orbital lipoma usually presents as a circumscribed orbital mass that has symptoms and signs similar to those of other circumscribed orbital tumors. Computed tomography and magnetic resonance imaging disclose a mass that may have heterogeneity or may have a consistency similar to orbital fat. The diagnosis usually is not made clinically, and the lipoma is recognized histopathologically after surgical excision.

SELECTED REFERENCES

1. Shields JA. *Diagnosis and management of orbital tumors.* Philadelphia: WB Saunders, 1989:234–236.
2. Johnson BL, Linn JG Fr. Spindle cell lipoma of the orbit. *Arch Ophthalmol* 1979;97:133–134.
3. Bartley GB, Yeatts RP, Garrity JA, Farrow GM, Campbell RJ. Spindle cell lipoma of the orbit. *Am J Ophthalmol* 1985;100:605–609.
4. Feinfield RE, Hesse RJ, Scharfenberg JC. Orbital angiolipoma. *Arch Ophthalmol* 1988;106:1093–1095.
5. Shields JA. *Diagnosis and management of orbital tumors.* Philadelphia: WB Saunders, 1989:238–239.

Lipoma

Orbital lipoma can assume any of several variations. Examples of a spindle cell lipoma, angiolipoma, and pleomorphic lipoma are shown. Another case of pleomorphic lipoma is shown in the *Atlas of Eyelid and Conjunctival Tumors*.

Figs. 9-13 and 9-14 courtesy of Dr. R. Jean Campbell. From Bartley GB, Yeatts RP, Garrity JA, Farrow GM, Campbell RJ. Spindle cell lipoma of the orbit. *Am J Ophthalmol* 1985;100:605–609.

Figs. 9-15 through 9-17 courtesy of Dr. Richard J. Hess. From Feinfield RE, Hesse RJ, Scharfenberg JC. Orbital angiolipoma. *Arch Ophthalmol* 1988;106:1093–1095.

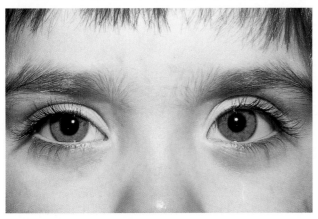

Figure 9-13. Spindle cell lipoma of the orbit. Coronal computed tomography of a 27-year-old man with a 7-year history of progressive fullness of the left upper eyelid.

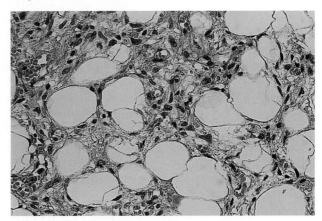

Figure 9-14. Histopathology of the lesion shown in Fig. 9-13 revealing mature lipocytes and uniform spindle cells (hematoxylin–eosin, original magnification × 160).

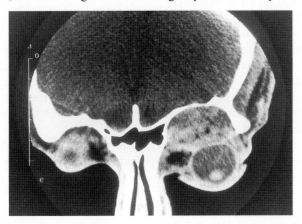

Figure 9-15. Angiolipoma of the orbit. Fullness of the left lower eyelid in a 3-year-old girl.

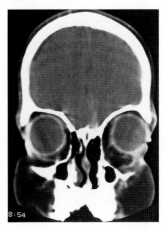

Figure 9-16. Coronal computed tomography of the child shown in Fig. 9-15 demonstrating low-density mass inferior to the left eye.

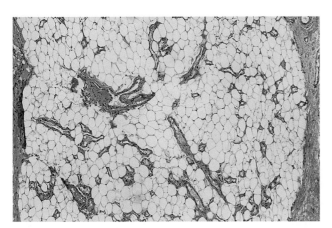

Figure 9-17. Histopathology of the lesion shown in Fig. 9-16 demonstrating lobules of adipose tissue with foci of microvascular proliferation (hematoxylin–eosin, original magnification × 100).

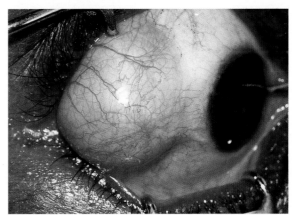

Figure 9-18. Pleomorphic lipoma of conjunctiva and orbit. Appearance of soft-yellow–pink mass in superotemporal quadrant in a 53-year-old man. Histopathology demonstrated a pleomorphic lipoma.

LIPOSARCOMA

Liposarcoma is a malignant tumor of adipose tissue. It is the most common soft-tissue sarcoma of adults. It is most common in the thigh, retroperitoneum, and inguinal region, but it has a widespread distribution. It occasionally occurs in the orbital region where is begins as a slow-growing circumscribed tumor that may be indistinguishable from other circumscribed orbital tumors (1,2). One small series indicated that the tumor usually involved the lateral rectus muscle (2).

Microscopically, liposarcomas have been divided into well-differentiated, myxoid, round-cell, and pleomorphic types. Most orbital liposarcomas are of the myxoid type and are called myxoid liposarcomas. It consists of fairly well-differentiated spindle, stellate, or round lipoblasts suspended in a myxoid or mucopolysaccharide-rich matrix, with a complex vascular system. This is in contrast to a pure myxoma, which shows a sparsity of vessels. Liposarcoma probably does not arise from a preexisting lipoma, but it probably develops from pluripotential mesenchymal cells that have the capacity toward lipocytic differentiation.

The best management of orbital liposarcoma is complete surgical excision. In advanced cases, orbital exenteration may be necessary. Irradiation can be employed for recurrent or completely excised tumors.

SELECTED REFERENCES

1. Shields JA. *Diagnosis and management of orbital tumors.* Philadelphia: WB Saunders, 1989:239–241.
2. Jakobiec FA, Rini F, Char D, Orcutt J, Rootman J, Baylis H, Flanagan J. Primary liposarcoma of the orbit. Problems in the diagnosis and management of five cases. *Ophthalmology* 1989;96:180–191.

Liposarcoma

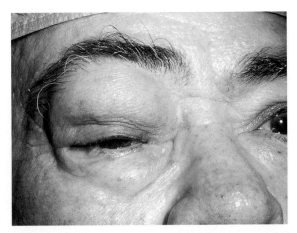

Figure 9-19. Extensive swelling of the right upper eyelid in a 78-year-old man. (Courtesy of Dr. Charles Lee.)

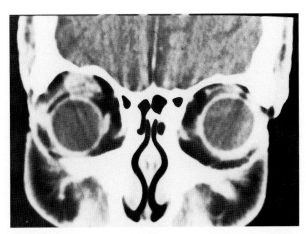

Figure 9-20. Coronal computed tomography of the patient shown in Fig. 9-19 demonstrating ovoid mass superior to the globe (Courtesy of Dr. Charles Lee.)

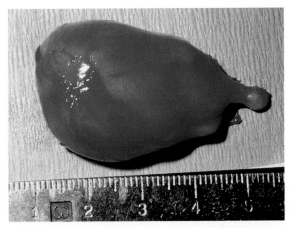

Figure 9-21. Gross appearance of the mass shown in Fig. 9-20 after excision. (Courtesy of Dr. Charles Lee.)

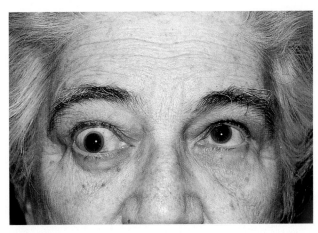

Figure 9-22. Proptosis of the right eye in an elderly woman. (Courtesy of Dr. Ralph C. Eagle Jr.)

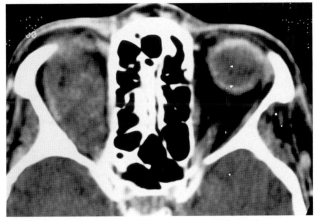

Figure 9-23. Axial computed tomography of the patient shown in Fig. 9-22 revealing ovoid mass filling most of posterior orbit. (Courtesy of Dr. Ralph C. Eagle Jr.)

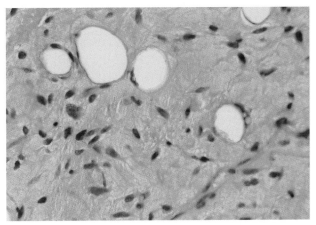

Figure 9-24. Histopathology of the lesion shown in Fig. 9-23 demonstrating tumor spindle cells in a myxomatous matrix (hematoxylin–eosin, original magnification × 100). (Courtesy of Dr. Ralph C. Eagle Jr.)

CHAPTER 10

Histiocytic Tumors and Pseudotumors

JUVENILE XANTHOGRANULOMA

Proliferative disorders of histiocytes comprise a spectrum of conditions ranging from solitary benign inflammatory processes to widely disseminated lesions that may exhibit malignant behavior. The general classification and current terminology for these disorders are discussed in more detail elsewhere (1). Conditions to be considered here include juvenile xanthogranuloma, Langerhan's cell histiocytosis, Erdheim–Chester disease, sinus histiocytosis with massive lymphadenopathy, and multinucleate cell angiohistiocytoma. Necrobiotic xanthogranuloma, a related condition, was discussed in the *Atlas of Eyelid and Conjunctival Tumors*.

Juvenile xanthogranuloma is a cutaneous eruption characterized by papules that develop in infants and young children. It has a rapid onset and progression, and then undergoes spontaneous resolution. It occasionally can affect the ocular structures, and it is also discussed in the *Atlas of Eyelid and Conjunctival Tumors*. Orbital involvement with juvenile xanthogranuloma is relatively rare, and it usually occurs as a solitary mass that can cause proptosis and displacement of the globe (1–3). Imaging studies show an irregular mass that usually is located in the anterior orbital structures. The diagnosis often is not made clinically, but it is made histopathologically after incisional or excisional biopsy. It is characterized histopathologically by a proliferation mainly of histiocytes with lymphocytes, plasma cells, eosinophils, and typical Touton giant cells, which stain positive for lipid. Electron microscopy generally does not show Birbeck granules, structures that characterize the Langerhan's cells seen with Langerhan's cell histiocytosis. The treatment is complete excision and systemic corticosteroids for recalcitrant cases. Irradiation generally is not warranted.

SELECTED REFERENCES

1. Shields JA. *Diagnosis and management of orbital tumors.* Philadelphia: WB Saunders, 1989:384–385.
2. Gaynes PM, Cohen GS, Juvenile xanthogranuloma of the orbit. *Am J Ophthalmol* 1967;63:755–757.
3. Shields CL, Shields JA, Buchanon H. Solitary orbital involvement with juvenile xanthogranuloma. *Arch Ophthalmol* 1990;108:1587–1589.

Juvenile Xanthogranuloma

Juvenile xanthogranuloma can occur as a solitary orbital mass in infants. A clinicopathologic correlation is illustrated.

From Shields CL, Shields JA, Buchanon H. Solitary orbital involvement with juvenile xanthogranuloma. *Arch Ophthalmol* 1990;108:1587–1589.

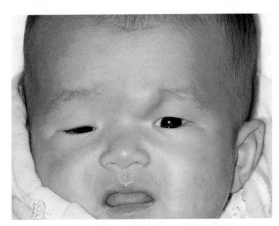

Figure 10-1. Subcutaneous mass superonasal to the left eye secondary to juvenile xanthogranuloma in a 3-month-old girl. The mass was noted at birth and had shown gradual enlargement.

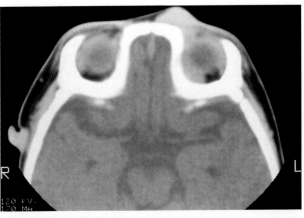

Figure 10-2. Axial computed tomography showing a solid mass extending posteriorly along the superonasal wall of the orbit.

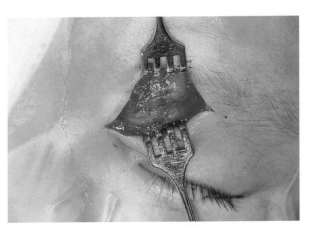

Figure 10-3. A biopsy of the subcutaneous portion of the mass was taken through a superonasal skin incision.

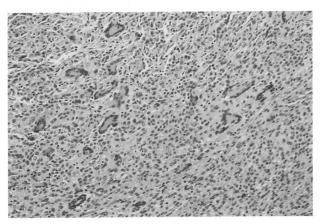

Figure 10-4. Histopathology showing sheets of histiocytes, chronic inflammatory cells, and giant cells (hematoxylin–eosin, original magnification × 50).

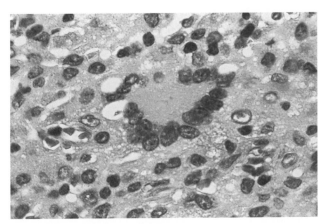

Figure 10-5. Histopathology showing giant cell with some lipid. It was classified as an atypical Touton giant cell (hematoxylin–eosin, original magnification × 250).

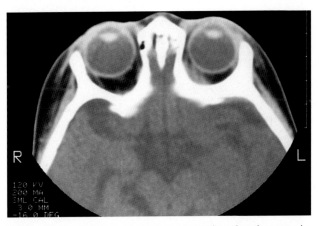

Figure 10-6. Axial computed tomography showing resolution of the orbital mass after a course of systemic corticosteroids.

LANGERHAN'S CELL HISTIOCYTOSIS (EOSINOPHILIC GRANULOMA)

Langerhan's cell histiocytosis is the currently accepted name for the histiocytosis X diseases, eosinophilic granuloma, Hand–Schuller–Christian disease, and Letterer–Siwe disease. The electron microscopic finding of cytoplasmic Birbeck granules, distinctive rod-shaped or tennis racquet–shaped structures, suggests that the Langerhan's cell is involved in the disease process. The most important of these with regard to the orbit is eosinophilic granuloma, which generally occurs in the orbital region as a solitary lesion of bone.

Eosinophilic granuloma usually has typical clinical features. It generally occurs in the first decade of life as a subacute swelling in the superotemporal aspect of the orbit, often with pain, redness, and tenderness over the bone superotemporally (1–3). In such cases, it can resemble a ruptured dermoid cyst, dacryoadenitis, or idiopathic orbital inflammation ("inflammatory pseudotumor"). It occasionally can develop in other quadrants and in the deeper orbital tissues. It occasionally is bilateral. Computed tomography and magnetic resonance imaging disclose an irregular, enhancing, bone destructive lesion in the zygomatic and/or frontal bones often with fragments of bone in the soft-tissue mass. Radiographically, it can resemble metastatic neuroblastoma, which occurs in somewhat younger children. Management includes biopsy with possible frozen sections to exclude the possibility followed by prompt and surgical curettage. Systemic or local corticosteroids can be employed (4). Cytotoxic agents or low-dose radiotherapy rarely are necessary. The lesion has a tendency to heal spontaneously without treatment (5).

SELECTED REFERENCES

1. Shields JA. *Diagnosis and management of orbital tumors.* Philadelphia: WB Saunders, 1989:378–382.
2. Feldman RB, Moore DM, Hood CI, Hiles DA, Romano PE. Solitary eosinophilic granuloma of the lateral orbital wall. *Am J Ophthalmol* 1985;100:318–323.
3. Jordan DR, McDonald H, Noel L, Nizalik E. Eosinophilic granuloma. *Arch Ophthalmol* 1993;111:134–135.
4. Wirtschafter JD, Nesbit M, Anderson P, McClain K. Intralesional methylprednisolone for Langerhan's cell histiocytosis of the orbit and cranium. J *Pediatr Ophthalmol Strabismus* 1987;14:195–197.
5. Glover AT, Grove AS. Eosinophilic granuloma of the orbit with spontaneous healing. *Ophthalmology* 1987;94:1008–1012.

Langerhan's Cell Histiocytosis (Eosinophilic Granuloma)— Clinical, Radiographic, and Pathologic Features

Fig. 10-12 courtesy of Dr. David Jordan. From Jordan DR, McDonald H, Noel L, Nizalik E. Eosinophilic granuloma. *Arch Ophthalmol* 1993;111:134–135.

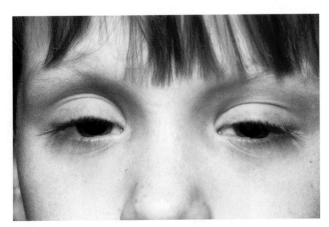

Figure 10-7. Eosinophilic granuloma. Swelling and blepharoptosis of the left upper eyelid in a 6-year-old boy.

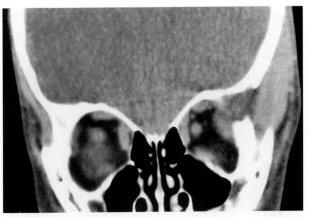

Figure 10-8. Coronal computed tomography of the patient shown in Fig. 10-7 demonstrating superotemporal bone destructive lesion with extension into the temporal fossa.

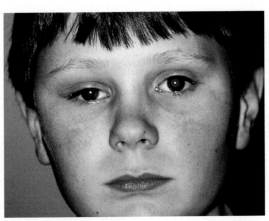

Figure 10-9. Eosinophilic granuloma. Swelling of the temporal fossa and slight blepharoptosis of the right upper eyelid in an 8-year-old boy.

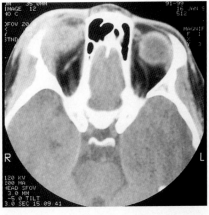

Figure 10-10. Axial computed tomography of the patient shown in Fig. 10-9 depicting mass in the lateral aspect of the orbit and temporal fossa with minor bone destruction.

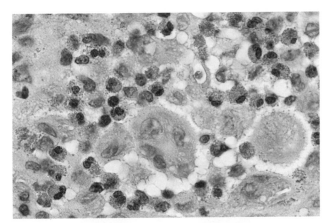

Figure 10-11. Histopathology of eosinophilic granuloma showing admixture of eosinophils, histiocytes, and giant cells (hematoxylin–eosin, original magnification × 200).

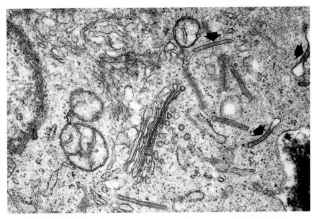

Figure 10-12. Electron photomicrograph showing characteristic Birbeck granules (*arrows*) in the cytoplasm of a histiocyte, a characteristic feature of Langerhan's cells (original magnification × 55,000).

Langerhan's Cell Histiocytosis (Eosinophilic Granuloma)—Management

In some cases, spontaneous healing can occur. A patient who underwent a biopsy for eosinophilic granuloma and subsequently healed spontaneously without additional treatment is depicted.

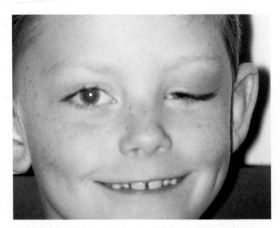

Figure 10-13. Redness and swelling superotemporal to the right eye in a 7-year-old boy.

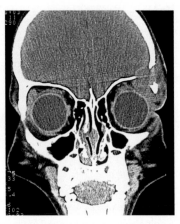

Figure 10-14. Coronal computed tomography with bone window showing large superotemporal bone destructive lesion.

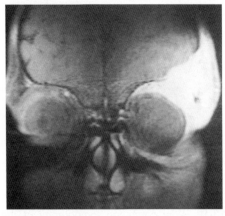

Figure 10-15. Coronal magnetic resonance imaging with gadolinium enhancement and fat suppression demonstrating enhancement of the mass.

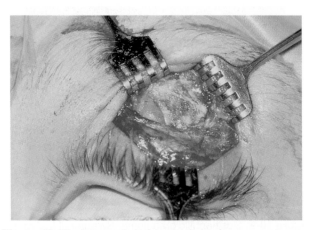

Figure 10-16. Approach to biopsy through a superotemporal cutaneous incision. Eosinophilic granuloma was diagnosed, and the patient was treated with systemic corticosteroids.

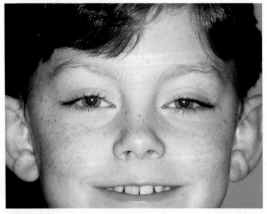

Figure 10-17. Appearance of the patient 1 year later showing marked improvement in appearance.

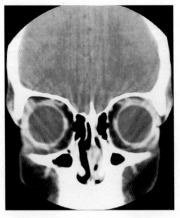

Figure 10-18. Coronal computed tomography 1 year later showing almost complete healing of the previously destroyed bone.

Langerhan's Cell Histiocytosis (Eosinophilic Granuloma)—Bilateral Sequential Orbital Involvement

In rare instances, bilateral sequential orbital involvement can occur. A case of bilateral orbital involvement with spontaneous healing is illustrated.

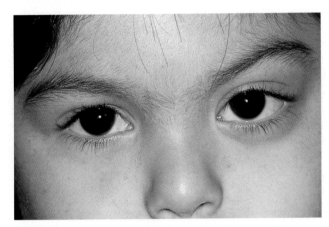

Figure 10-19. Anterior orbital mass causing superotemporal fullness above the left eye in a 5-year-old boy.

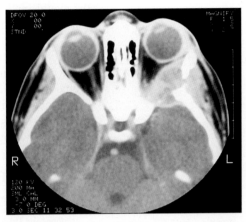

Figure 10-20. Axial computed tomography showing bone destructive mass involving orbit and temporal fossa. A biopsy and curettage was done.

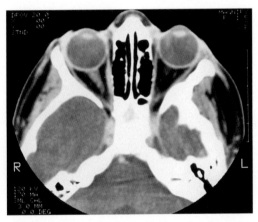

Figure 10-21. Axial computed tomography done 6 months later showing almost complete resolution of the mass and remodeling of the bone.

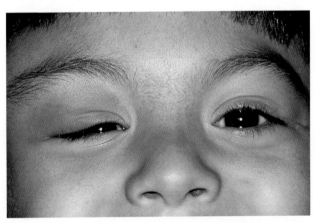

Figure 10-22. Appearance of the child 18 months after initial presentation showing acute involvement superotemporally in the right orbit.

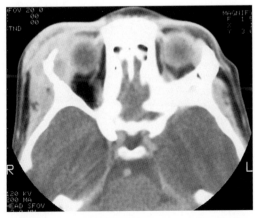

Figure 10-23. Axial computed tomography done at the same time as Fig. 10-22 demonstrating soft tissue and bone involvement in the right orbit. The left orbit has mostly healed, but there is hyperostosis.

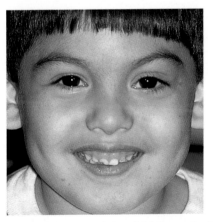

Figure 10-24. Appearance of the child 6 months later after both orbits had healed spontaneously demonstrating marked improvement in facial appearance.

ERDHEIM–CHESTER DISEASE

Erdheim–Chester disease is a peculiar form of systemic xanthogranulomatosis that is characterized by infiltration of many organs including lung, kidney, heart, bones, retroperitoneal tissue, and occasionally the orbit (1–4). It tends to occur in adulthood, and the orbital involvement usually is bilateral. It is characterized by xanthelasma of the eyelids and bilateral proptosis. Imaging studies show diffuse orbital masses that sometimes can fill the entire orbital cavity. Although the disease often affects long bones, the orbital involvement is usually in soft tissue, without significant bone involvement. Massive soft-tissue infiltration can lead to marked proptosis and optic-nerve compression with visual loss in one or both eyes. Imaging studies show diffuse orbital masses. Histopathologically, there is a diffuse infiltration of the affected tissues by histiocytes with chronic inflammatory cells and occasional Touton giant cells. Most treatments are not highly effective, but systemic corticosteroids, cytotoxic agents, or radiotherapy may be attempted (1–4).

SELECTED REFERENCES

1. Shields JA. *Diagnosis and management of orbital tumors.* Philadelphia: WB Saunders, 1989:385.
2. Alper MG, Zimmerman LE, LaPiana FG. Orbital manifestations of Erdheim–Chester disease. *Trans Am Ophthalmol Soc* 1983;891:64–85.
3. Shields JA, Karcioglu Z, Shields CL, Eagle RC Jr, Wong S. Orbital and eyelid involvement with Erdheim–Chester disease. *Arch Ophthalmol* 1991;109:850–854.
4. Valmaggia C, Neuweiler J, Fretz C, Gottlob I. A case of Erdheim–Chester disease with orbital involvement. *Arch Ophthalmol* 1997;115:1467–1468.

Erdheim–Chester Disease

Erdheim–Chester disease characterized by bilateral xanthelasmas and bilateral proptosis. These findings should arouse suspicion of the diagnosis. The orbital involvement is often massive. Two brief cases are illustrated.

From Shields JA, Karcioglu Z, Shields CL, Eagle RC Jr, Wong S. Orbital and eyelid involvement with Erdheim–Chester disease. *Arch Ophthalmol* 1991;109:850–854.

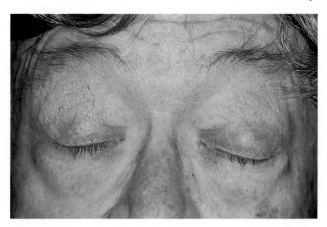

Figure 10-25. Xanthelasma on both upper eyelids in a 78-year-old man with bilateral proptosis and systemic findings of Erdheim–Chester disease, including pulmonary and retroperitoneal fibrosis.

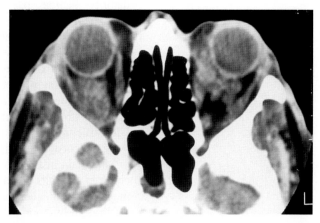

Figure 10-26. Axial computed tomography of the patient shown in Fig. 10-25 demonstrating patchy involvement of both orbits by soft-tissue infiltration.

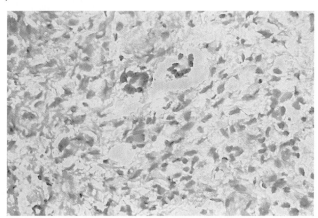

Figure 10-27. Histopathology of orbital biopsy from the left eye of the patient shown in Fig. 10-25 demonstrating infiltration of histiocytes and Touton giant cells (hematoxylin–eosin, original magnification × 150).

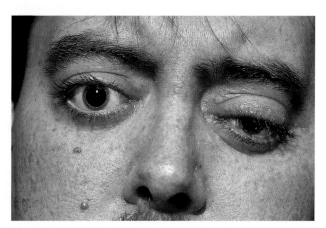

Figure 10-28. Bilateral proptosis and atypical xanthelasmas in a 28-year-old man. The patient had severe visual loss in both eyes secondary to massive orbital involvement and optic-nerve compression.

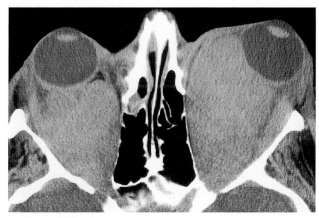

Figure 10-29. Axial computed tomography of the patient shown in Fig. 10-28 demonstrating massive infiltration of both orbits.

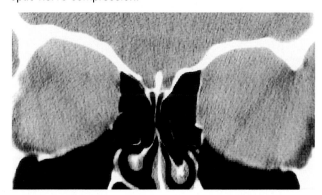

Figure 10-30. Coronal computed tomography of the patient shown in Fig. 10-28 further demonstrating the extent of the orbital involvement.

SINUS HISTIOCYTOSIS, MALIGNANT HISTIOCYTOSIS, AND MULTINUCLEATE CELL ANGIOHISTIOCYTOMA

Miscellaneous other histiocytic lesions that can involve the orbit, either as a solitary lesion or as a part of widespread systemic involvement, include sinus histiocytosis, malignant histiocytosis, and multinucleate cell angiohistiocytoma.

Sinus histiocytosis with massive lymphadenopathy (Rosai–Dorfman disease) is a distinct benign pseudolymphomatous entity with characteristic clinical and histopathologic features (1,2). This idiopathic condition is characterized by extensive lymph node enlargement, particularly the cervical nodes. The word sinus in the title refers to the sinus of lymph nodes and not the paranasal sinuses. Orbital involvement occurs in approximately 10% of cases, in which cases it appears as unilateral or bilateral infiltration of soft tissues (3). It is more common in young black males. Histopathology shows a polymorphous infiltration of mature lymphocytes with histiocytes that often contain phagocytosed lymphocytes, plasma cells, and erythrocytes. Ultrastructural studies fail to show Birbeck granules. The disease is self-limited, but systemic corticosteroids and low-dose radiotherapy may have a role in severe cases.

Malignant histiocytosis appears to be a true malignancy of histiocytes. It occurs in children or adults who may present with fever, anemia, leukopenia, and hepatosplenomegaly. It can occur as a diffuse orbital mass. Histopathologically, there is a diffuse infiltration by poorly differentiated malignant histiocytes. The disease is often fatal, but some patients have shown good remission with intensive chemotherapy (4).

Multinucleate cell angiohistiocytoma is an idiopathic, benign vascular condition characterized clinically by multiple, grouped, violaceous, nonpainful, cutaneous papules that generally occur in the extremities of women over the age of 40 years. It recently has been diagnosed in the orbit as a circumscribed anterior orbital mass (5). Histopathologically, it is characterized by increased numbers of small blood vessels in the dermis, a sparse lymphocytic infiltration, histiocytes, and prominent multinucleated giant cells. Immunohistochemical studies have indicated that the dermal cells are compatible with histiocytes. The pathogenesis is uncertain.

SELECTED REFERENCES

1. Shields JA. *Diagnosis and management of orbital tumors.* Philadelphia: WB Saunders, 1989:378–388.
2. Friendly DS, Font RL, Rao NA. Orbital involvement in "sinus" histiocytosis. A report of four cases. *Arch Ophthalmol* 1977;95:2006–2011.
3. Foucar E, Rosai J, Dorfman RF. The ophthalmologic manifestations of sinus histiocytosis with massive lymphadenopathy. *Am J Ophthalmol* 1979;87:354–367.
4. Takahashi T, Katsumori N, Urano Y, et al. A case of malignant histiocytosis. *Ophthalmologica* 1984;188:159–164.
5. Shields JA, Eagle RC Jr, Shields CL, Sohmer KK. Multinucleate cell angiohistiocytoma of the orbit. *Am J Ophthalmol* 1995;120:402–403.

Sinus Histiocytosis, Malignant Histiocytosis, and Multinucleate Cell Angiohistiocytoma

Figs. 10-34 through 10-36 from Shields JA, Eagle RC Jr, Shields CL, Sohmer KK. Multinucleate cell angiohistiocytoma of the orbit. *Am J Ophthalmol* 1995;120:402–403.

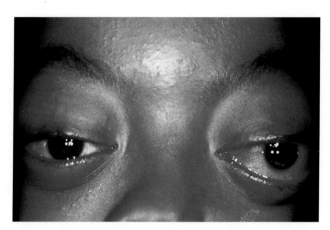

Figure 10-31. Orbital involvement by sinus histiocytosis. Typical clinical appearance of bilateral proptosis in a young male. (Courtesy of Dr. Narsing Rao.)

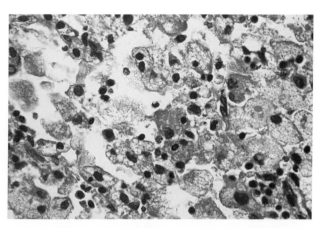

Figure 10-32. Histopathology of sinus histiocytosis showing histiocytes that have phagocytosed lymphocytes and erythrocytes (hematoxylin–eosin, original magnification × 200). (Courtesy of Dr. John Gamel.)

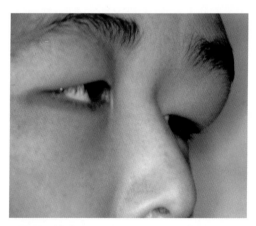

Figure 10-33. Malignant histiocytosis. Extensive superior orbital involvement in a young adult male. (Courtesy of Dr. Toshihiro Takahashi.)

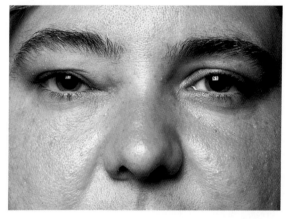

Figure 10-34. Multinucleate cell angiohistiocytoma. Superonasal anterior orbital mass in a 38-year-old woman. There were no extraocular lesions.

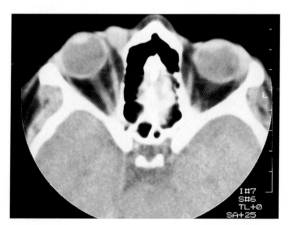

Figure 10-35. Axial computed tomography of the patient shown in Fig. 10-34 demonstrating a circumscribed anterior orbital mass.

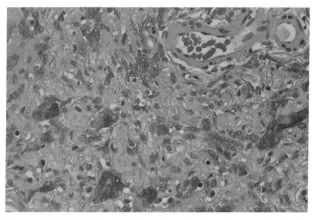

Figure 10-36. Histopathology showing blood vessels, histiocytes, and characteristic multinucleated giant cells, typical of multinucleate cell angiohistiocytoma (hematoxylin–eosin, original magnification × 200).

CHAPTER 11

Primary Melanocytic Tumors

ORBITAL MELANOMA ARISING FROM BLUE NEVUS

Primary melanocytic tumors of the orbit include melanoma, melanocytic hamartoma, and melanotic neuroectodermal tumor of infancy (retinal anlage tumor). Primary orbital melanoma usually arises from congenital orbital melanocytosis or orbital congenital blue nevus (1). Examples of orbitopalpebral melanoma arising from blue nevus in the anterior aspect of the orbit were shown in the *Atlas of Eyelid and Conjunctival Tumors*.

Most primary orbital melanomas arise from congenital cellular blue nevus (1–4) or from congenital ocular melanocytosis (1–6). In some cases, the underlying orbital cellular blue nevus is subclinical and does not produce symptoms until it spawns a melanoma later in life. In other cases, the cellular blue nevus appears as an episcleral or subconjunctival pigmentation similar to typical ocular melanocytosis, except that it may be more elevated rather than flat. The melanoma that arises from either of these congenital conditions generally is circumscribed, even though the underlying congenital pigmentation is diffuse and not circumscribed. Proptosis in a patient with either congenital ocular melanocytosis or blue nevus should arouse suspicion of a primary orbital melanoma or orbital extension of a uveal melanoma.

Imaging studies can detect the circumscribed orbital mass and help, along with clinical examination, to exclude the possibility of a uveal melanoma. Because the melanoma usually is well circumscribed, an attempt should be made to remove the tumor intact by excisional biopsy. The surrounding flat congenital pigmentation should be examined at surgery, biopsied, and treated with heavy cryotherapy. An incisional biopsy of a circumscribed orbital mass in the setting of congenital ocular melanocytosis generally is contraindicated and complete removal is preferable. Orbital melanoma can recur locally and can metastasize to distant organs if it is not controlled locally.

SELECTED REFERENCES

1. Shields JA. *Diagnosis and management of orbital tumors.* Philadelphia: WB Saunders, 1989:279–282.
2. Shields JA. Orbital malignant melanomas. In: Hornblass A, ed. *Ophthalmic plastic and reconstructive surgery.* Baltimore: Williams & Wilkins, 1988:1048–1052.
3. Gunduz K, Shields JA, Shields CL, Eagle RC Jr. Periorbital cellular blue nevus leading to orbitopalpebral and intracranial melanoma. *Ophthalmology* 1998;105:2046–2050.
4. Tellado M, Specht CS, McLean IW, Grossniklaus HE, Zimmerman LE. Primary orbital melanoma. *Ophthalmology* 1996;103:929–932.
5. Dutton JJ, Anderson RL, Schleper RL, Purcell JJ, Tse DT. Orbital malignant melanoma and oculodermal melanocytosis. Report of two cases and review of the literature. *Ophthalmology* 1984;91:497–507.
6. Wilkes SR, Uthman EO, Thornton CN, et al. Malignant melanoma of the orbit in a black patient with ocular melanocytosis. *Arch Ophthalmol* 1984;102:904–906.

Orbital Melanoma Arising from Blue Nevus

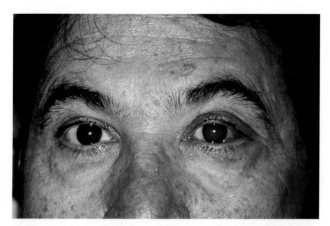

Figure 11-1. Proptosis of the left eye in a 59-year-old man who had thick congenital ipsilateral epibulbar pigmentation temporally. The proptosis was of recent onset and associated with epibulbar hyperemia, suggestive of an inflammatory process.

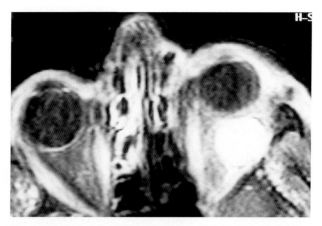

Figure 11-2. Axial orbital magnetic resonance imaging with gadolinium enhancement in T1-weighted image of the patient shown in Fig. 11-1. Note the circumscribed mass temporal to the optic nerve. At the time of surgery, marked pigmentation was found throughout the temporal portion of the orbit, including the sheath of the lateral rectus muscle.

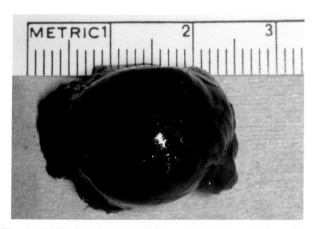

Figure 11-3. Appearance of the orbital mass shown in Fig. 11-2 after surgical removal.

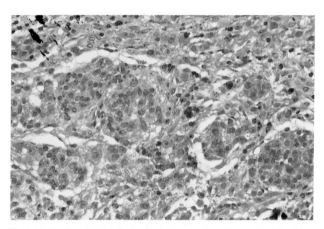

Figure 11-4. Histopathology of the lesion shown in Fig. 11-3 demonstrating lobules of spindle- and epithelioid cell melanoma. Biopsy of adjacent tissues demonstrated cellular blue nevus.

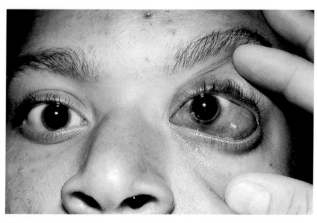

Figure 11-5. Black patient with ocular melanocytosis with an orbitoconjunctival nodule of recent onset. (Courtesy of Dr. David Wilkes.)

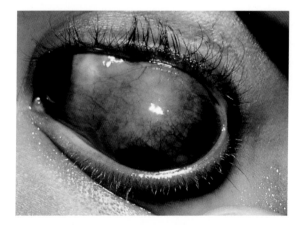

Figure 11-6. Closer view of the lesion shown in Fig. 11-5. The lesion was excised and proved to be a malignant melanoma. (Courtesy of Dr. David Wilkes.)

ORBITAL MELANOMA ARISING *DE NOVO*

In some instances, orbital melanoma apparently arises *de novo* without clinical evidence of preexisting ocular melanocytosis or blue nevus (1–3). It is possible that such congenital rests of pigment were present but were subclinical. However, even detailed histopathologic studies have failed to reveal an underlying pigmentary process. The tumor is generally circumscribed. The diagnosis often is not made clinically, but it can be suspected at surgery when a circumscribed solid black tumor is detected.

It is important to remove an orbital melanoma intact by way of an excisional biopsy. A cutaneous and systemic evaluation should be done to exclude an occult primary melanoma that could have metastasized to the orbit.

SELECTED REFERENCES

1. Shields JA. *Diagnosis and management of orbital tumors.* Philadelphia: WB Saunders, 1989:279–282.
2. Shields JA. Orbital malignant melanomas. In: Hornblass A, ed: *Ophthalmic plastic and reconstructive surgery.* Baltimore: Williams & Wilkins, 1988:1048–1052.
3. Shields JA, Shields CL, Eagle RC Jr, De Potter P, Oliver GL. Necrotic orbital melanoma arising de novo. *Br J Ophthalmol* 1993;77:187–189.

Orbital Melanoma Arising *De Novo*

In some instances, an orbital melanoma appears to arise when there is no apparent congenital melanosis. A clinicopathologic correlation of a necrotic primary orbital melanoma is shown.

From Shields JA, Shields CL, Eagle RC Jr, De Potter P, Oliver GL. Necrotic orbital melanoma arising de novo. *Br J Ophthalmol* 1993;77:187–189.

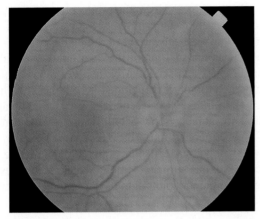

Figure 11-7. Fundus photograph of the right eye showing optic disc edema in a 76-year-old man who complained of blurred vision.

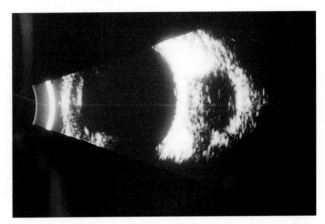

Figure 11-8. B-scan ultrasonogram showing round, acoustically hollow retrobulbar mass.

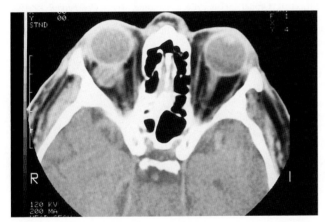

Figure 11-9. Axial computed tomography showing a circumscribed intraconal right retrobulbar mass. The mass was removed via a conjunctival approach.

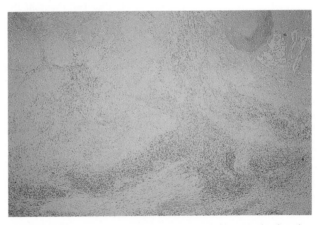

Figure 11-10. Low-magnification photomicrograph showing massive necrosis in the central portion of the tumor (hematoxylin–eosin, original magnification × 20).

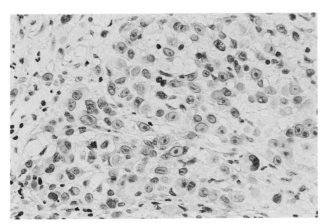

Figure 11-11. Section through a peripheral portion of the mass showing spindle and epithelioid melanoma cells (hematoxylin–eosin, original magnification × 200).

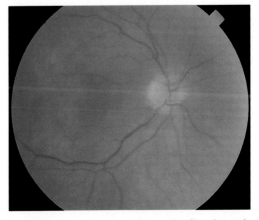

Figure 11-12. Appearance of the optic disc 6 weeks after surgery showing resolution of the optic disc edema.

MELANOCYTIC HAMARTOMA AND MELANOTIC NEUROECTODERMAL TUMOR

Rare primary melanocytic tumors of the orbit include the melanocytic hamartoma and the neuroectodermal tumor of infancy (1). A giant melanocytic hamartoma has been described in the orbit of a newborn. The mass was present at birth and covered the anterior aspect of the orbit, filling the palpebral aperture and obscuring the globe. Pathologically, it encased the globe as a solid pigmented mass and diffusely involved the uveal tract (2). Histopathologically, the tumor cells in the orbit were spindle shaped and dendritic and those in the uveal tract were round, similar to a melanocytoma. This poorly understand tumor may represent an unusual variant of a blue nevus (2).

Melanotic neuroectodermal tumor is an unusual tumor that is often congenital and begins in the maxillary or zygomatic bones and secondarily involves the orbital soft tissue. Because it is a primary pigmented tumor, it is included here rather than in the chapter on secondary tumors. It occurs in infancy as a secondary orbital mass that can displace the globe. Imaging studies presumably show a lytic lesion of the affected bones with secondary soft-tissue involvement in the orbit. Histopathologically, it is composed of glandular tubules lined by polygonal cells that contain pigment. The cells are separated by abundant connective tissue stroma. Although the pathogenesis is uncertain, the close similarity to retinal pigment epithelium has prompted some investigators to use the term retinal anlage tumor (3–5).

SELECTED REFERENCES

1. Shields JA. *Diagnosis and management of orbital tumors.* Philadelphia: WB Saunders, 1989:279–282.
2. Char DH, Crawford JB, Ablin AR, et al. Orbital melanocytic hamartoma. *Am J Ophthalmol* 1981;91: 357–361.
3. Hall WC, O'Day DM, Glick AD. Melanotic neuroectodermal tumor of infancy. An ophthalmic appearance. *Arch Ophthalmol* 1979;97:922–925.
4. Halpert B, Pratzer R. Maxillary tumor of retinal anlage. *Surgery* 1947;22:837–841.
5. Koudstaal J, Oldhoff J, Panders AK, et al. Melanotic neuroectodermal tumor of infancy. *Cancer* 1968; 22:151–161.

Melanocytic Hamartoma and Melanotic Neuroectodermal Tumor

Figs. 11-13 through 11-15 courtesy of Drs. Deveron Char and Brooks Crawford. From Char DH, Crawford JB, Ablin AR, et al. Orbital melanocytic hamartoma. *Am J Ophthalmol* 1981;91:357–361.

Figs. 11-16 through 11-18 courtesy of Dr. Devron O'Day. From Hall WC, O'Day DM, Glick AD. Melanotic neuroectodermal tumor of infancy. An ophthalmic appearance. *Arch Ophthalmol* 1979;97:922–925.

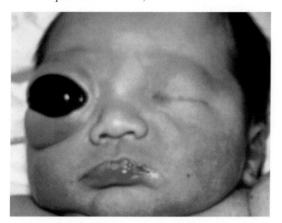

Figure 11-13. Giant melanocytic hamartoma of the orbit in an Asian infant. Note the extensive pigmented mass filling the palpebral aperture.

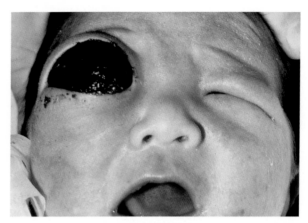

Figure 11-14. Another view of the lesion shown in Fig. 11-13.

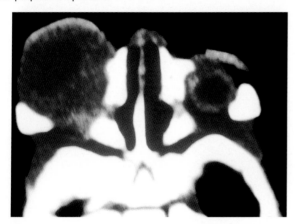

Figure 11-15. Axial computed tomography of the lesion shown in Fig. 11-13 showing larger right orbit secondary to orbital mass.

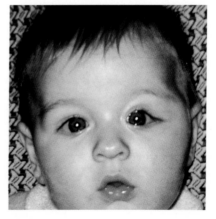

Figure 11-16. Melanotic neuroectodermal tumor of infancy. Medial displacement of the globe in an infant secondary to a lateral orbital mass.

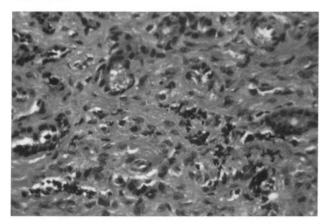

Figure 11-17. Histopathology showing tubules and acini of pigment epithelial cells separated by a connective tissue stroma (hematoxylin–eosin, original magnification × 100).

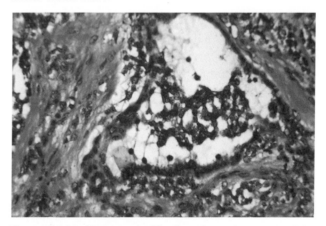

Figure 11-18. Higher-magnification photomicrograph of the lesion shown in Fig. 11-17 (hematoxylin–eosin, original magnification × 100).

CHAPTER 12

Epithelial Tumors of the Lacrimal Gland

DACRYOPS

Important epithelial lesions of the lacrimal gland include dacryops, pleomorphic adenoma, and malignant epithelial tumors (1,2). In a review of 142 consecutive biopsies of lacrimal gland masses, 22% were epithelial lesions and 78% were nonepithelial lesions, mainly inflammations and lymphoid tumors (3).

Dacryops (lacrimal ductal cyst) is a cyst of the lacrimal gland. In a review of 645 orbital biopsies, it accounted for 5 cases (less than 1%). In the review of 142 lacrimal gland biopsies, it accounted for 6% of cases. The frequency is probably higher, because most lesions are relatively small and do not come to surgical excision.

Dacryops usually arises from the palpebral lobe of the lacrimal gland in adults and presents as a painless, nontender, fluctuant mass in the forniceal conjunctiva superotemporally (1,4–6). It can occur spontaneously or it can follow dacryoadenitis. It is often slowly progressive, but it can remain stable for long periods of time. Imaging studies demonstrate a cystic mass corresponding to the anterior part of the lacrimal gland, In contrast to dermoid cyst and malignant lacrimal gland tumor, there are usually no fossa or bone destruction. Histopathologically, it is a cystic lesion with a clear lumen and an epithelial lining that consists of one or two layers of somewhat flattened epithelium, similar to a lacrimal gland duct. Smaller asymptomatic lesions can be observed, and large ones can be resected locally by a superotemporal conjunctival forniceal approach, taking care not to disrupt the ducts that drain the palpebral lobe if possible.

SELECTED REFERENCES

1. Shields JA. *Diagnosis and management of orbital tumors.* Philadelphia: WB Saunders, 1989:260–262.
2. Shields JA, Bakewell B, Augsburger DG, Flanagan CJ. Classification and incidence of space-occupying lesions of the orbit. A survey of 645 biopsies. *Arch Ophthalmol* 1984;102:1606–1611.
3. Shields CL, Shields JA, Eagle RC Jr, Rathmell JP. Clinicopathologic review of 142 cases of lacrimal gland lesions. *Ophthalmology* 1989;96:431–435.
4. Brownstein S, Belin MW, Krohel GB, et al. Orbital dacryops. *Ophthalmology* 1984;91:1424–1428.
5. Bullock JD, Fleishman JA, Rosset JS. Lacrimal ductal cysts. *Ophthalmology* 1986;93:1355–1360.
6. Smith S, Rootman J. Lacrimal ductal cysts. Presentation and management. *Surv Ophthalmol* 1986;30:245–250.

Dacryops

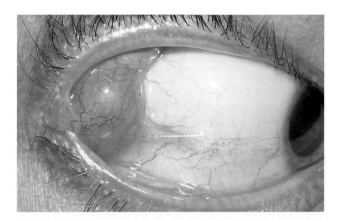

Figure 12-1. Dacryops superotemporally in a 55-year-old man. The lesion was producing persistent discomfort.

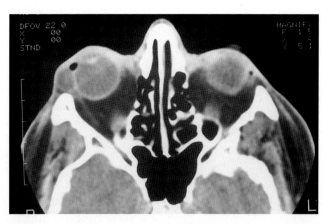

Figure 12-2. Axial computed tomography of the patient shown in Fig. 12-1 demonstrating a cystic lesion near the anterior orbital rim.

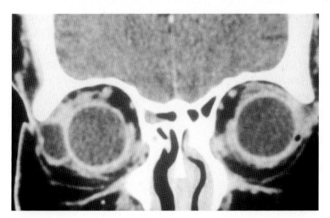

Figure 12-3. Coronal computed tomography showing a cystic lesion temporal to the globe.

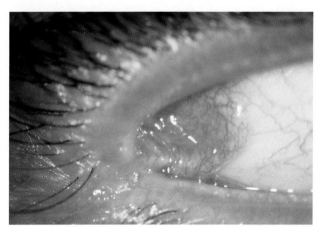

Figure 12-4. Appearance of the intact lesion at the time of surgical removal by a superotemporal conjunctival approach.

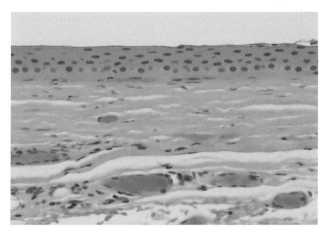

Figure 12-5. Histopathology showing flattened epithelium and fibrous tissue wall of the cyst.

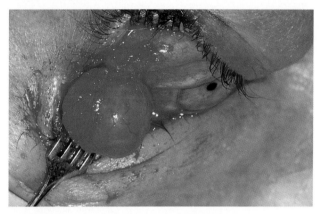

Figure 12-6. Appearance 5 months later showing no recurrence. The patient's symptoms resolved.

PLEOMORPHIC ADENOMA (BENIGN MIXED TUMOR)

Pleomorphic adenoma is the most important benign epithelial tumor of the lacrimal gland (1–6). In the author's series of orbital biopsies, it accounted for greater than 2% of 645 specimens (2). Among 142 lacrimal gland biopsies, it accounted for 12% of cases (3). Series in which the cases are collected strictly from a tumor clinic show a higher incidence of pleomorphic adenoma (4). It usually arises from the orbital lobe of the lacrimal gland. Most cases occur in adults as a unilateral progressive nonpainful mass in the anterior aspect of the orbit superotemporally. As the lesion enlarges, it typically produces proptosis and downward and nasal displacement of the globe. Imaging studies disclose a round to ovoid circumscribed mass with a smooth to slightly irregular surface. There may be fossa formation in the adjacent bone but frank bone destruction, as seen with some malignant tumors, usually is not evident. Computed tomography is the best method to assess bone involvement (7).

The histopathologic features of pleomorphic adenoma vary from case to case. The most typical feature is a combination of benign epithelial elements and mesenchymal elements, accounting for the name benign mixed tumor. The epithelial elements can take the form of ducts, cords, and squamous pearls. The mesenchymal elements usually include myxoid and chondroid tissue. If the diagnosis of pleomorphic adenoma of the lacrimal gland is suspected on the basis of clinical findings and imaging studies, the tumor should be removed by a superolateral orbitotomy through an eyelid crease incision with an extraperiosteal approach. An osteotomy (Kronlein approach) is not necessary in most cases. It generally is mandatory to excise completely the mass in its capsule without a prior biopsy. Incisional biopsy may hinder complete tumor removal and allow for recurrence and possible malignant transformation. With time, pleomorphic adenoma can evolve into pleomorphic adenocarcinoma (malignant mixed tumor) (8).

SELECTED REFERENCES

1. Shields JA. *Diagnosis and management of orbital tumors.* Philadelphia: WB Saunders, 1989:265–267.
2. Shields JA, Bakewell B, Augsburger DG, Flanagan CJ. Classification and incidence of space-occupying lesions of the orbit. A survey of 645 biopsies. *Arch Ophthalmol* 1984;102:1606–1611.
3. Shields CL, Shields JA, Eagle RC Jr, Rathmell JP. Clinicopathologic review of 142 cases of lacrimal gland lesions. *Ophthalmology* 1989;96:431–435.
4. Reese AB. Expanding lesions of the orbit. Bowman Lecture. *Trans Ophthalmol Soc UK* 1971;91:85–104.
5. Shields JA, Shields CL, Eagle RC Jr, Rizzo J. Pleomorphic adenoma ("benign mixed tumor") of the lacrimal gland. *Arch Ophthalmol* 1987;105:560–561.
6. Wright JE, Stewart WB, Krohel GB. Clinical presentation and management of lacrimal gland tumours. *Br J Ophthalmol* 1979;63:600–606.
7. Jakobiec FA, Trokel SL, Abbott GF, et al. Combined clinical and computed tomographic diagnosis of primary lacrimal fossa lesions. *Am J Ophthalmol* 1982;94:785–807.
8. Shields JA, Shields CL. Malignant transformation of presumed pleomorphic adenoma of lacrimal gland after 60 years. *Arch Ophthalmol* 1987;105:1403–1405.

Pleomorphic Adenoma of the Lacrimal Gland—Clinicopathologic Correlation

From Shields JA, Shields CL, Eagle RC Jr, Rizzo J. Pleomorphic adenoma ("Benign mixed tumor") of the lacrimal gland. *Arch Ophthalmol* 1987;105:560–561.

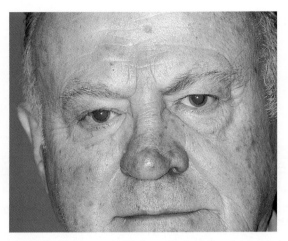

Figure 12-7. Downward displacement of the right eye in a 73-year-old man.

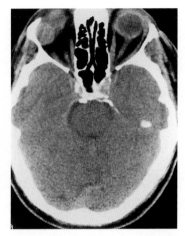

Figure 12-8. Axial computed tomography showing an ovoid mass in the lacrimal gland fossa.

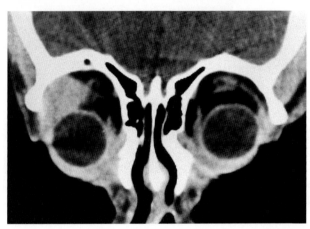

Figure 12-9. Coronal computed tomography showing the same lesion.

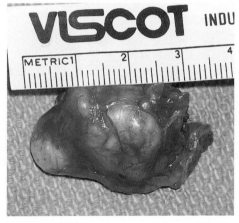

Figure 12-10. Gross appearance of the mass after successful surgical removal. Note the lobular surface of the encapsulated mass.

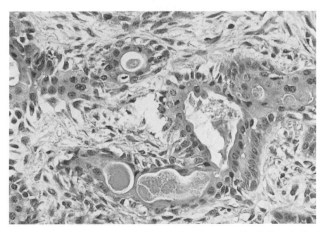

Figure 12-11. Histopathology showing epithelial tubules within myxomatous stroma (hematoxylin–eosin, original magnification × 100).

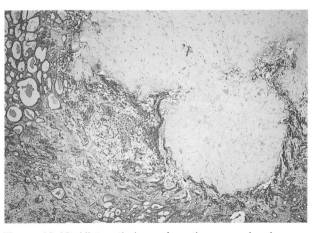

Figure 12-12. Histopathology of another area showing cartilaginous differentiation (hematoxylin–eosin, original magnification × 50).

Pleomorphic Adenoma of the Lacrimal Gland—Surgical Management

The goal of treatment is to remove the tumor intact through a superolateral orbitotomy, usually without an osteotomy.

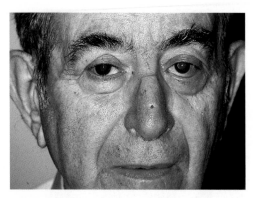

Figure 12-13. Proptosis and downward displacement of the left eye in a 71-year-old man.

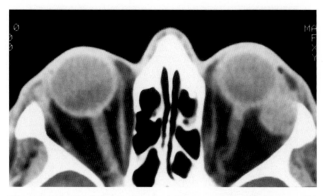

Figure 12-14. Axial computed tomography showing solid, round mass in superotemporal aspect of orbit anteriorly.

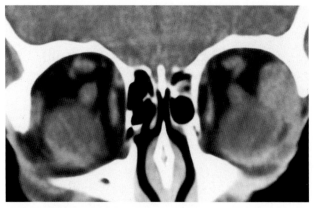

Figure 12-15. Coronal computed tomography showing ovoid mass superotemporal to the globe.

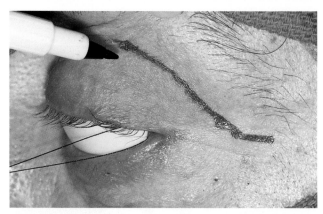

Figure 12-16. Outlined incision to perform tumor removal through a superotemporal cutaneous eyelid crease approach.

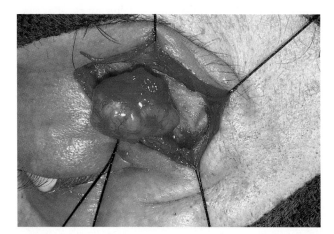

Figure 12-17. Appearance of the tumor as it is being removed.

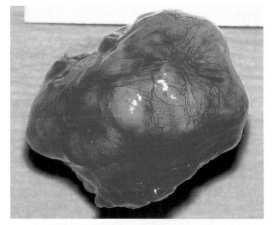

Figure 12-18. Gross appearance of encapsulated mass. Note the characteristic light-yellow color and the nodularity of the margin of the lesion.

Pleomorphic Adenoma of the Lacrimal Gland in a Young Patient

Pleomorphic adenoma of the lacrimal gland generally appears in middle-aged or older patients. Occasionally it can develop in a younger patient. A clinicopathologic correlation is shown.

From Mercado G, Gunduz K, Shields JA, Shields CL, Eagle RC Jr. Pleomorphic adenoma of the lacrimal gland in a young patient. *Arch Ophthalmol* 1998;116:962–963.

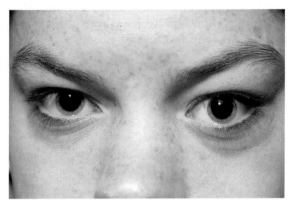

Figure 12-19. Proptosis secondary to a superotemporal orbital mass in a 15-year-old girl.

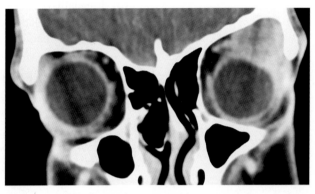

Figure 12-20. Coronal computed tomography showing mass in lacrimal gland fossa. Note that the slow-growing lesion has produced marked superior displacement of the frontal and zygomatic bones.

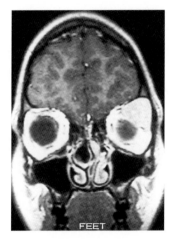

Figure 12-21. Coronal magnetic resonance imaging in T1-weighted image showing triangular-shaped enhancing solid mass.

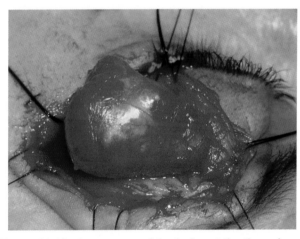

Figure 12-22. Appearance of the lesion at the time of successful surgical removal.

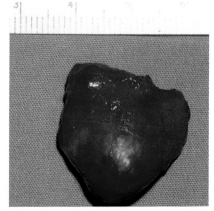

Figure 12-23. Gross appearance of encapsulated mass. Note the characteristic surface nodularity of the lesion.

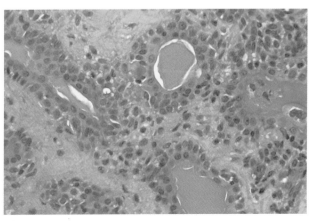

Figure 12-24. Histopathology showing epithelial and mesenchymal elements characteristic of pleomorphic adenoma.

PLEOMORPHIC ADENOCARCINOMA (MALIGNANT MIXED TUMOR)

Malignant epithelial tumors of the lacrimal gland are aggressive neoplasms (1). Although several types have been identified, the most important are pleomorphic adenocarcinoma (malignant mixed tumor) and adenoid cystic carcinoma.

Pleomorphic adenocarcinoma can occur from malignant transformation of a pleomorphic adenoma, particularly if the benign lesion was excised incompletely (2,3). It accounted for three cases (2%) of the 142 lacrimal gland lesions in the author's series (4). It usually occurs in older patients, and imaging studies show a large orbital mass arising from the lacrimal gland fossa, often with bone erosion. The management is the same as for adenoid cystic carcinoma described subsequently.

SELECTED REFERENCES

1. Shields JA. *Diagnosis and management of orbital tumors.* Philadelphia: WB Saunders, 1989:267–272.
2. Henderson JW, Farrow GM. Primary malignant mixed tumors of the lacrimal gland. Report of 10 cases. *Ophthalmology* 1980;17:466–475.
3. Shields JA, Shields CL. Malignant transformation of presumed pleomorphic adenoma of lacrimal gland after 60 years. *Arch Ophthalmol* 1987;105:1403–1405.
4. Shields CL, Shields JA, Eagle RC Jr, Rathmell JP. Clinicopathologic review of 142 cases of lacrimal gland lesions. *Ophthalmology* 1989;96:431–435.

Pleomorphic Adenocarcinoma of the Lacrimal Gland

Pleomorphic adenocarcinoma can evolve from a preexisting pleomorphic adenoma of the lacrimal gland after many years. A clinicopathologic correlation is shown.

From Shields JA, Shields CL. Malignant transformation of presumed pleomorphic adenoma of lacrimal gland after 60 years. *Arch Ophthalmol* 1987;105:1403–1405.

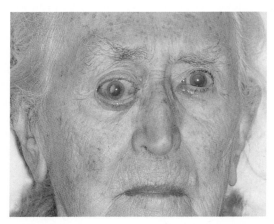

Figure 12-25. Proptosis of the right eye in an 81-year-old woman. Mild proptosis had been noted 60 years earlier, and the diagnosis of a benign lacrimal gland tumor was made but no treatment was given. The previously stable proptosis had increased progressively for 18 months.

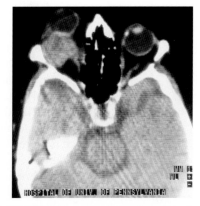

Figure 12-26. Axial computed tomography showing large mass in the lacrimal gland fossa causing severe proptosis. Biopsy under local anesthesia revealed pleomorphic adenoma, but the patient declined further surgery because of her advanced age and poor cardiovascular status. Orbital radiation was given.

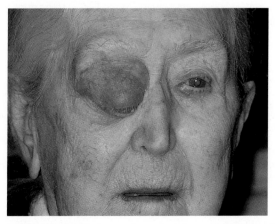

Figure 12-27. Appearance 3 years later when the patient developed tumor recurrence with worsening of the proptosis. A protective tarsorrhaphy had been performed.

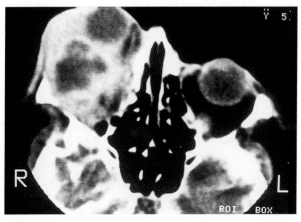

Figure 12-28. Axial computed tomography showing massive tumor recurrence. The patient agreed to orbital exenteration.

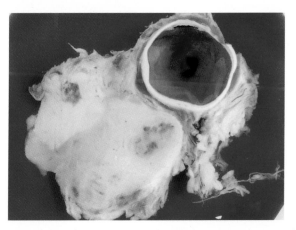

Figure 12-29. Gross section of orbital exenteration specimen showing globe (*top*) and massive orbital tumor.

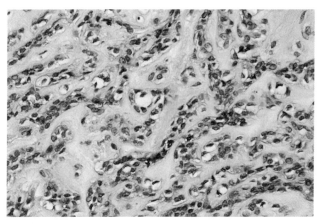

Figure 12-30. Histopathology showing cords of malignant epithelial cells in a myxoid stroma (hematoxylin–eosin, original magnification × 100).

ADENOID CYSTIC CARCINOMA OF THE LACRIMAL GLAND

Adenoid cystic carcinoma is the best known of the malignant epithelial neoplasms of the lacrimal gland (1–5). Although it accounted for only two cases (1%) of the lacrimal gland biopsies in the author's earlier series (3), several cases have been identified since that time, and it may be more common than indicated by that series. Although it usually is diagnosed in middle-aged or older patients, it frequently occurs in younger patients as well (6–8). A recent study suggested that young patients with this tumor may have a more favorable prognosis (7). The affected patient frequently develops pain because of the tendency of this tumor to invade nerves. Adenoid cystic carcinoma has also been known to arise in the nasal orbit, distant from the main lacrimal gland (9). Histopathologically, adenoid cystic carcinoma can assume any of several patterns, the best known of which is the typical cystic spaces lined by malignant cells, the so-called "Swiss cheese" pattern. The basaloid pattern is said to impart the worse prognosis (10). If the tumor is circumscribed, it can be removed entirely. If it is more extensive, a biopsy should be done; if the diagnosis is confirmed histopathologically, orbital exenteration with removal of affected bone should be done. Supplemental radiation and chemotherapy should be considered in advanced cases. In some cases, local brachytherapy using a radioactive plaque had been used, but there is no long-term follow-up of this method. It is possible that earlier detection with computed tomography or magnetic resonance imaging may allow more efficient treatment and a better prognosis in the future.

SELECTED REFERENCES

1. Shields JA. *Diagnosis and management of orbital tumors.* Philadelphia: WB Saunders, 1989:267–272.
2. Henderson JW, Farrow GM. Primary malignant mixed tumors of the lacrimal gland. Report of 10 cases. *Ophthalmology* 1980;17:466–475.
3. Shields CL, Shields JA, Eagle RC Jr, Rathmell JP. Clinicopathologic review of 142 cases of lacrimal gland lesions. *Ophthalmology* 1989;96:431–435.
4. Font RL, Gamel JW. Adenoid cystic carcinoma of the lacrimal gland. A clinicopathologic study of 79 cases. In: Nicholson DH, ed. *Ocular pathology update.* New York: Masson, 1980:277–283.
5. Lee DA, Campbell RJ, Waller RR, Ilstrup DM. A clinicopathologic study of primary adenoid cystic carcinoma of the lacrimal gland. *Ophthalmology* 1985;92:128–134.
6. Dagher G, Anderson RL, Ossoinig KC, Baker JD. Adenoid cystic carcinoma of the lacrimal gland in a child. *Arch Ophthalmol* 1980;98:1098–1100.
7. Tellado MV, McLean IW, Specht CS, Varga J. Adenoid cystic carcinomas of the lacrimal gland in childhood and adolescence. *Ophthalmology* 1997;104:1622–1625.
8. Shields JA, Shields CL, Eagle RC Jr, Freire JE, Mercado GV, Schnall B. Adenoid cystic carcinona of the lacrimal gland in a 9-year-old child. *Arch Ophthalmol* 1998;116:1673–1676.
9. Shields JA, Shields CL, Eagle RC Jr, Adkins J, De Potter P. Adenoid cystic carcinoma arising in the nasal orbit. *Am J Ophthalmol* 1997;123:398–399.
10. Gamel JW, Font RL. Adenoid cystic carcinoma of the lacrimal gland. The clinical significance of a basaloid histologic pattern. *Hum Pathol* 1982;13:219–225.

Adenoid Cystic Carcinoma of the Lacrimal Gland

Adenoid cystic carcinoma of the lacrimal has characteristic clinical and radiographic features. Management often requires orbital exenteration and irradiation. A clinical course and clinicopathologic correlation is shown.

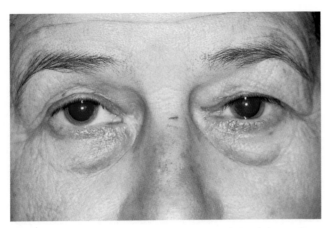

Figure 12-31. Downward displacement of the left eye in a 57-year-old woman.

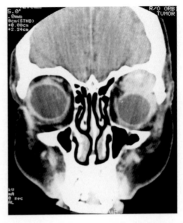

Figure 12-32. Coronal computed tomography showing orbital mass arising in the lacrimal gland fossa. Note that there are characteristic densities that suggest calcium, a finding seen in many adenoid cystic carcinomas.

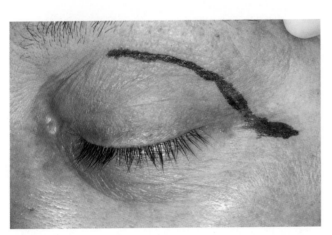

Figure 12-33. Planned surgical approach by a superotemporal orbitotomy with a cutaneous eyelid crease incision.

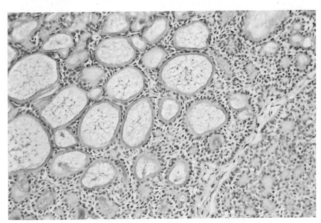

Figure 12-34. Histopathology showing Swiss cheese pattern of adenoid cystic carcinoma (hematoxylin–eosin, original magnification × 100).

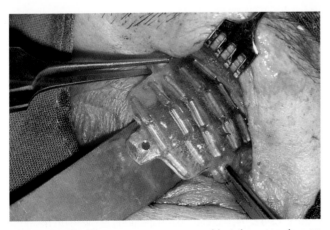

Figure 12-35. The tumor was removed but the capsule was invaded by adenoid cystic carcinoma. Therefore, brachytherapy was employed using a custom-designed radioactive iodine-125 plaque, which is being placed in the superotemporal aspect of the orbit.

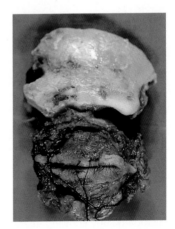

Figure 12-36. After 6 years, there was a recurrence in the roof of the orbit and frontal sinus. Combined orbital exenteration and removal of frontal sinus was done. Shown are the orbital contents (*bottom*) and the frontal bone (*top*) removed in one piece.

Adenoid Cystic Carcinoma of the Lacrimal Gland

Adenoid cystic carcinoma of the lacrimal has a tendency to occur in young children as well as in adults. A clinicopathologic correlation and management of such a case in a 9-year-old boy is depicted.

From Shields JA, Shields CL, Eagle RC Jr, Freire JE, Mercado GV, Schnall B. Adenoid cystic carcinona of the lacrimal gland in a 9-year-old child. *Arch Ophthalmol* 1998;116:1673–1676.

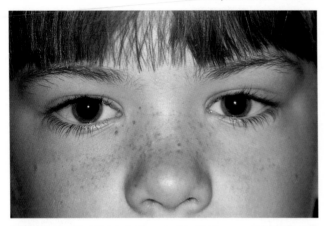

Figure 12-37. Minimal downward displacement of the left eye in a 9-year-old boy who complained of headaches.

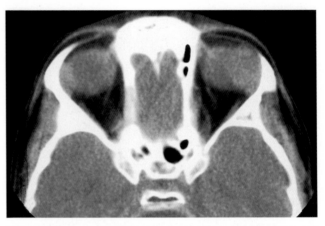

Figure 12-38. Axial computed tomography showing a round superotemporal orbital mass.

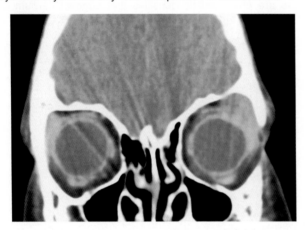

Figure 12-39. Coronal computed tomography showing bony fossa formation from the mass. This pattern raised suspicion of a chronic benign lesion.

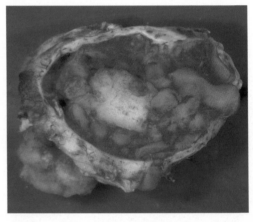

Figure 12-40. Section of the gross specimen after surgical removal by a superolateral orbitotomy. The yellow central material raised suspicion of a dermoid cyst based on gross observation.

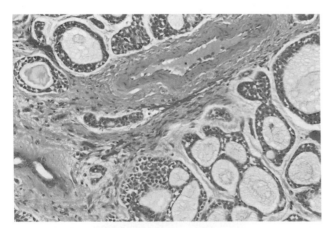

Figure 12-41. Histopathology showing adenoid cystic carcinoma (hematoxylin–eosin, original magnification × 100).

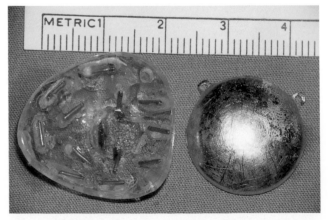

Figure 12-42. Additional frozen sections showed no residual orbital tumor and the visual acuity was perfect, so the patient was treated with brachytherapy using a radioactive plaque rather than orbital exenteration. Shown is the active plaque with I-125 seeds (*left*) and the gold shield placed over the sclera to protect the globe from the radiation.

Adenoid Cystic Carcinoma—Atypical Orbital Location

In rare instances, adenoid cystic carcinoma can occur in the orbit away from the lacrimal gland. The etiology of such a tumor is uncertain, but it is possible that it could develop from ectopic lacrimal gland. A case is illustrated.

From Shields JA, Shields CL, Eagle RC Jr, Adkins J, De Potter P. Adenoid cystic carcinoma arising in the nasal orbit. *Am J Ophthalmol* 1997;123:398–399.

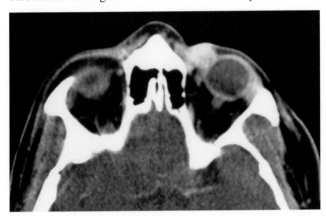

Figure 12-43. Axial computed tomography of a 27-year-old man showing a round mass in the nasal portion of the orbit anteriorly. The patient was managed elsewhere at this time by an incomplete biopsy, and the diagnosis of adenoid cystic carcinoma was made.

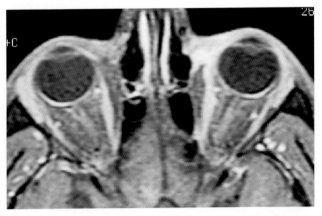

Figure 12-44. Axial magnetic resonance imaging shown 2 weeks later demonstrating enhancing tissue nasally suspicious of persistent tumor. Frozen sections revealed diffuse persistent tumor, and an eyelid-sparing orbital exenteration was performed.

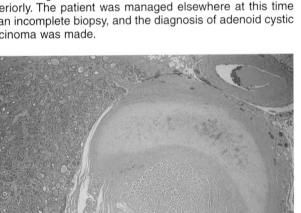

Figure 12-45. Histopathology of exenteration specimen showing adenoid cystic carcinoma adjacent to the trochlea.

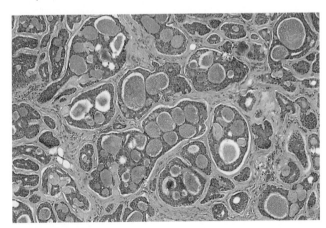

Figure 12-46. Histopathology showing adenoid cystic carcinoma (hematoxylin–eosin, original magnification × 75).

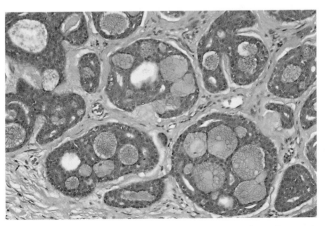

Figure 12-47. Histopathology showing adenoid cystic carcinoma (hematoxylin–eosin, original magnification × 150).

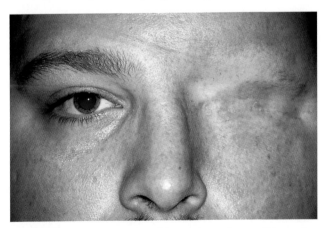

Figure 12-48. Appearance of the patient after eyelid-sparing exenteration showing good healing. A prosthesis was subsequently used with good cosmetic result.

CHAPTER 13

Metastatic Tumors
to the Orbit

ORBITAL METASTASIS

A metastatic cancer to the orbit is a malignant neoplasm that has spread to the orbit by way of the bloodstream (1–4). In adults, most tumors that metastasize to the orbit are carcinomas that arise from the epithelial structures of breast, prostate, lung, gastrointestinal tract, and other organs (1–7). In children, orbital metastases are more likely to arise from embryonal neural tumors and sarcomas, such as neuroblastoma, Wilms' tumor, and Ewing's tumor (8–11). Most patients with breast cancer metastasis to the orbit have a history of treated breast cancer. Many patients with metastasis from lung cancer or carcinoid tumor have no history of cancer, and the orbital mass may be the first sign of malignancy.

The patient with orbital metastasis may experience rapid onset of proptosis, displacement of the eye, pain, diplopia, and conjunctival and eyelid edema. Some scirrhous tumors can produce a paradoxical enophthalmos (7). Computed tomography and magnetic resonance imaging findings vary with the primary tumor. Metastatic breast cancer may be more diffuse and grow along fascial planes and muscle. Prostate metastasis tends to affect orbital bone. Metastatic melanoma, carcinoid tumor, and renal cell carcinoma may be very circumscribed, resembling a benign orbital tumor (8–10). The diagnosis generally should be confirmed by orbital biopsy. If there no known primary and no other metastasis, then an open biopsy should be done by the most accessible route as determined by imaging studies. If the patient has a known primary and possible metastasis elsewhere, then fine-needle aspiration biopsy may be warranted. Subsequent treatment with irradiation and chemotherapy generally is employed, depending on the clinical circumstances (1–4). Selected examples of orbital metastasis are shown.

SELECTED REFERENCES

1. Shields CL, Shields JA, Peggs M. Tumors metastatic to the orbit. *Ophthal Plast Reconstr Surg* 1988;4:73–80.
2. Goldberg RA, Rootman J, Cline RA. Tumors metastatic to the orbit: a changing picture. *Surv Ophthalmol* 1990;35:1–24.
3. Shields CL, Shields JA, Eagle RC Jr, Peyster RG, Conner BE, Green HA. Orbital metastasis from a carcinoid tumor. Computed tomography, magnetic resonance imaging, and electron microscopic findings. *Arch Ophthalmol* 1987;105:968–971.
4. Shields CL, Shields JA, Mruczek AW. Enophthalmos as the initial manifestation of metastasis from scirrhous carcinoma of the breast. *Ophthalmic Pract* 1989;7:159–160.
5. Shields JA, Shields CL, Brucker WK, Novak J. Metastatic renal cell carcinoma to the orbit. *Ophthalmic Pract* 1989;7:239–242.
6. Font RL, Naumann G, Zimmerman LE. Primary malignant melanoma of the skin metastatic to the eye and orbit. *Am J Ophthalmol* 1967;63:738–754.
7. Goldberg SH, Kennedy RE, Metz HS, Searl SS, Rose SJ. Strabismus caused by melanoma metastatic to an extraocular muscle. *Ann Ophthalmol* 1990;22:467–471.
8. Musarella M, Chan HSL, DeBoer G, et al. Ocular involvement in neuroblastoma. Prognostic implications. *Ophthalmology* 1984;91:936–940.
9. Fratkin D, Purcell JJ, Krachmer JH, et al. Wilms' tumor metastasis to the orbit. *JAMA* 1977;238:1841–1842.
10. Kawachi E, Nunobiki K, Shimada S, et al. A case of Ewing's sarcoma with orbital metastasis. *Folia Ophthalmol Jpn* 1984;35:1840–1845.
11. Fekrat S, Miller NR, Loury MC. Alveolar rhabdomyosarcoma that metastasized to the orbit. *Arch Ophthalmol* 1993;111:1662–1664.

Orbital Metastasis from Breast Cancer

Breast cancer accounts for the majority of orbital metastasis. It usually produces proptosis, with the exception of scirrhous breast cancer, which can contract, causing a paradoxical enophthalmos.

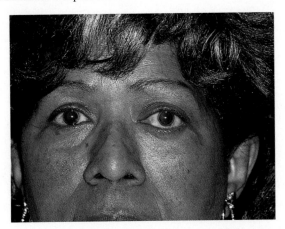

Figure 13-1. Proptosis of the left eye secondary to orbital metastasis from breast cancer in a 68-year-old woman.

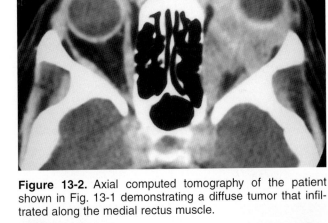

Figure 13-2. Axial computed tomography of the patient shown in Fig. 13-1 demonstrating a diffuse tumor that infiltrated along the medial rectus muscle.

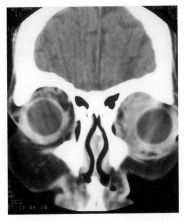

Figure 13-3. Coronal computed tomography of the patient shown in Fig. 13-1 demonstrating a diffuse tumor that encases the globe.

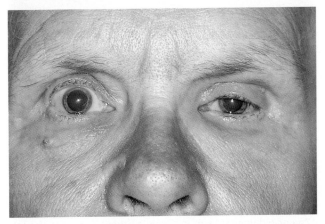

Figure 13-4. Enophthalmos of the left eye secondary to metastatic scirrhous breast cancer to the orbit in a 75-year-old woman. She was referred with the diagnosis of proptosis of the right eye, which proved to be normal.

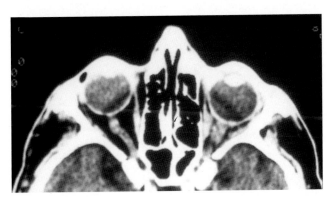

Figure 13-5. Axial computed tomography of the patient shown in Fig. 13-4. There is diffuse contracting tumor tissue in the medial and posterior orbit producing the enophthalmos.

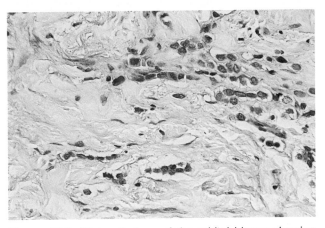

Figure 13-6. Histopathology of the orbital biopsy showing desmoplasia with cords of malignant tumor cells, characteristic of metastatic breast cancer (hematoxylin–eosin, original magnification × 100).

Orbital Metastasis from Breast Cancer—Clinical Variations

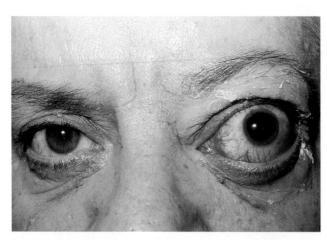

Figure 13-7. Unilateral proptosis and upward displacement of the left eye secondary to metastatic breast cancer in a 65-year-old woman.

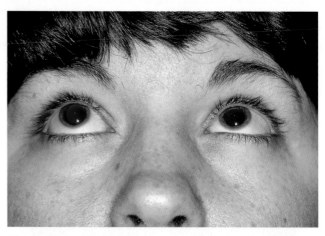

Figure 13-8. Slight limitation of upgaze of the left eye secondary to metastatic breast cancer to the left orbit in a 38-year-old woman.

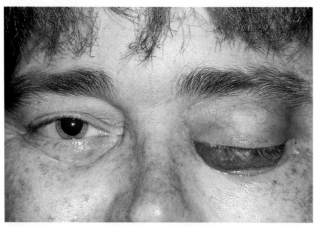

Figure 13-9. Blepharoptosis and conjunctival chemosis in a 47-year-old woman with metastatic breast cancer to the left orbit.

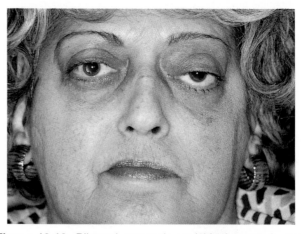

Figure 13-10. Bilateral proptosis and blepharoptosis secondary to bilateral orbital metastasis in a 64-year-old woman.

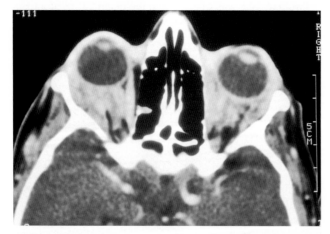

Figure 13-11. Axial computed tomography showing bilateral orbital metastasis from breast cancer. (Courtesy of Dr. Peter Rubin.)

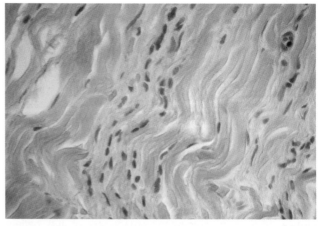

Figure 13-12. Histopathology of the orbital biopsy of the patient shown in Fig. 13-11 demonstrating fibrous tissue and cords of malignant tumor cells, characteristic of metastatic breast cancer (hematoxylin–eosin, original magnification × 100).

Orbital Metastasis from Breast Cancer—Biopsy Techniques

Depending on the clinical findings and the size and location of the tumor, either excisional biopsy, incisional biopsy, or fine-needle aspiration biopsy can be performed.

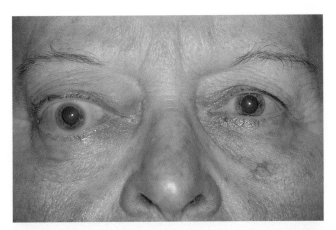

Figure 13-13. Proptosis of the right eye in a 76-year-old woman with breast cancer but no prior history of metastasis.

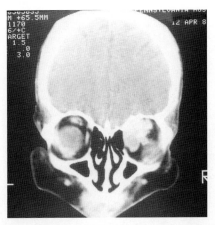

Figure 13-14. Coronal computed tomography of the patient shown in Fig. 13-13 showing mass in the superonasal aspect of the right orbit.

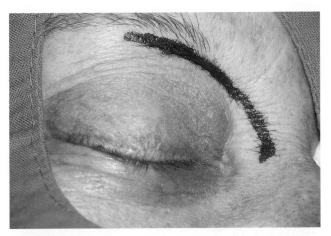

Figure 13-15. Planned superonasal cutaneous incision as determined by coronal computed tomography.

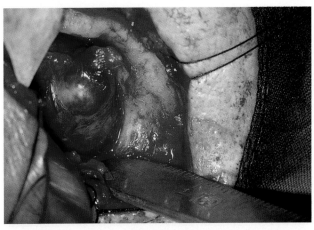

Figure 13-16. Tumor being removed intact by excisional biopsy.

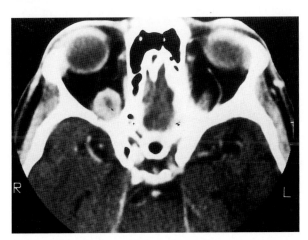

Figure 13-17. Posterior orbital metastasis in a 58-year-old woman. Coronal computed tomography showing a small tumor in the posterior aspect of the orbit. Careful computed tomography-guided, fine-needle aspiration biopsy was performed.

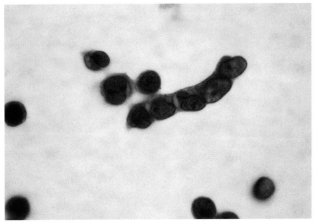

Figure 13-18. Cytology of fine-needle biopsy for orbital metastasis of breast cancer showing characteristic cells (Papanicolaou, original magnification × 250).

Orbital Metastasis from Prostate Carcinoma

Prostate cancer metastatic to the orbital area has a propensity to affect orbital bones more than soft tissue. Immunohistochemistry for prostate-specific antigen can assist in the histopathologic diagnosis.

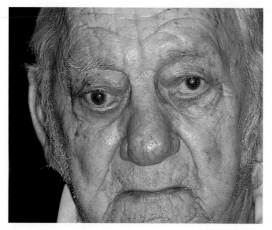

Figure 13-19. Proptosis and downward displacement of the right eye in a 79-year-old man with prostate cancer.

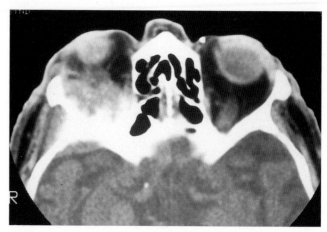

Figure 13-20. Axial computed tomography of the patient shown in Fig. 13-19 demonstrating extensive bone and soft-tissue involvement with metastatic prostate cancer.

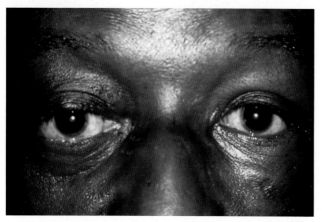

Figure 13-21. Downward displacement of the right eye in a 56-year-old man with prostate cancer.

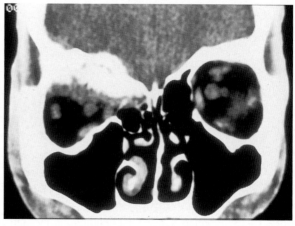

Figure 13-22. Coronal computed tomography of the patient shown in Fig. 13-21 demonstrating involvement of bone in the roof of the orbit and mild soft-tissue involvement.

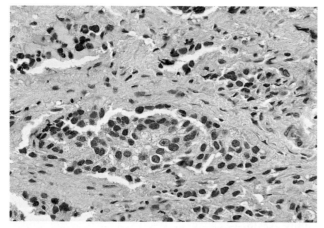

Figure 13-23. Histopathology of orbital biopsy from the patient shown in Fig. 13-21 demonstrating cells compatible with metastatic prostate cancer (hematoxylin–eosin, original magnification × 100).

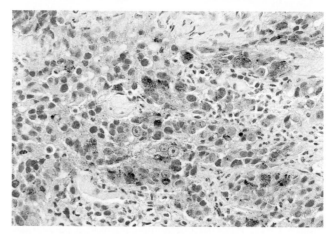

Figure 13-24. Immunohistochemistry for prostate-specific antigen of the specimen shown in Fig. 13-23 demonstrating immunopositivity (original magnification × 100).

Orbital Metastasis from Carcinoid Tumor

Ocular metastasis from bronchial carcinoid tumor usually involves the uveal tract. In contrast, ocular metastasis from ileal or appendiceal carcinoid tends to affect the orbit. The reason for these metastatic patterns is unknown. A clinicopathologic correlation of a carcinoid tumor of the ileum metastatic to the orbit is shown.

From Shields CL, Shields JA, Eagle RC Jr, Peyster RG, Conner BE, Green HA. Orbital metastasis from a carcinoid tumor. Computed tomography, magnetic resonance imaging, and electron microscopic findings. *Arch Ophthalmol* 1987;105:968–971.

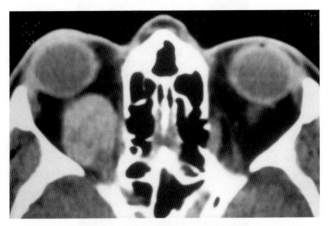

Figure 13-25. Axial computed tomography of a 63-year-old woman with a history of carcinoid tumor of the ileum who developed progressive proptosis of the right eye.

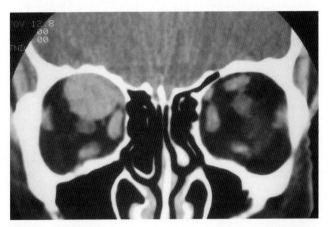

Figure 13-26. Coronal computed tomography showing superior orbital mass.

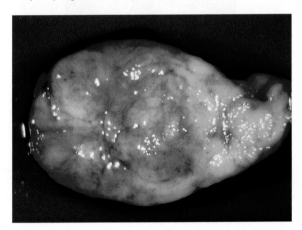

Figure 13-27. Gross appearance of resected tumor.

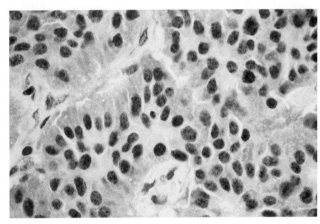

Figure 13-28. Histopathology showing large cells with prominent hyperchromatic eccentric nuclei and granular eosinophilic cytoplasm (hematoxylin–eosin, original magnification × 250).

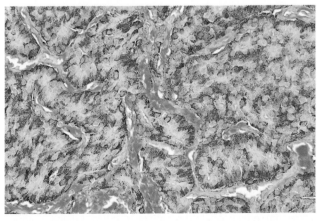

Figure 13-29. Histopathology showing argyrophilic neurosecretory granules (Grimelius, original magnification × 400).

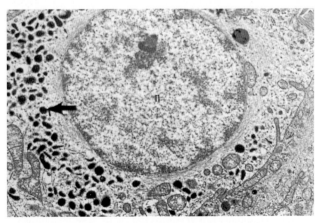

Figure 13-30. Electron photomicrograph showing carcinoid cell with large nucleus and neurosecretory granules in the cytoplasm (*arrow*) (original magnification × 14,000).

Orbital Metastasis from Lung Cancer and Thyroid Cancer

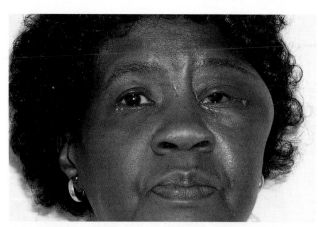

Figure 13-31. Proptosis and swelling of the temporal fossa secondary to metastatic lung cancer in a 57-year-old woman.

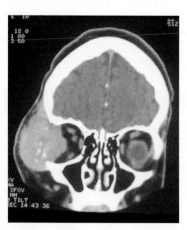

Figure 13-32. Coronal computed tomography of the patient shown in Fig. 13-31 demonstrating large bone-destructive tumor.

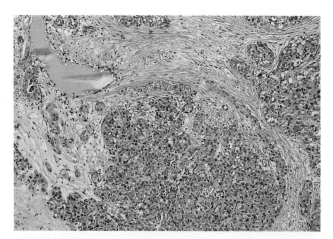

Figure 13-33. Orbital metastasis from Hurthle cell carcinoma of the thyroid gland. Proptosis and chemosis of the left eye in a 41-year-old woman. (Courtesy of Dr. R. Jean Campbell.)

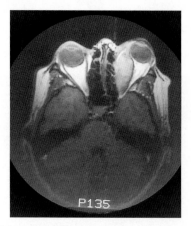

Figure 13-34. Axial magnetic resonance imaging in T1-weighted image of the patient shown in Fig. 13-33 showing fusiform mass in medial aspect of the orbit involving the medial rectus muscle. (Courtesy of Dr. R. Jean Campbell.)

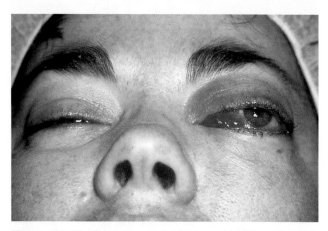

Figure 13-35. Histopathology of the lesion shown in Fig. 13-33 demonstrating nodule of tumor cells (hematoxylin–eosin, original magnification × 50). (Courtesy of Dr. R. Jean Campbell.)

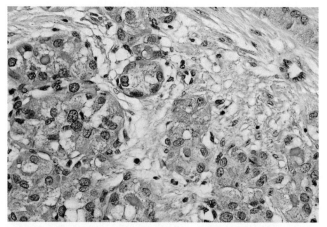

Figure 13-36. Histopathology showing solid lobule and acini of tumor cells. Immunohistochemical stains for thyroglobulin were markedly positive (hematoxylin–eosin, original magnification × 150). (Courtesy of Dr. R. Jean Campbell.)

Orbital Metastasis from Renal Cell Carcinoma and Melanoma

Figs. 13-37 through 13-39 from Shields JA, Shields CL, Brucker WK, Novak J. Metastatic renal cell carcinoma to the orbit. *Ophthalmic Pract* 1989;7:239–242.

Figs. 13-40 through 13-42 courtesy of Dr. Steven Searl. From Goldberg SH, Kennedy RE, Metz HS, Searl SS, Rose SJ. Strabismus caused by melanoma metastatic to an extraocular muscle. *Ann Ophthalmol* 1990;22:467–471.

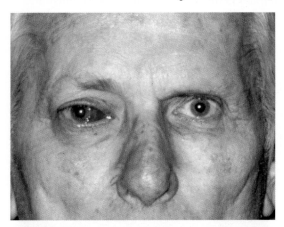

Figure 13-37. Metastatic renal cell carcinoma to the orbit. Proptosis and lateral displacement of the right eye in a 68-year-old man with a history of renal cell carcinoma but no known metastasis. The conjunctival redness is due to a prior biopsy done elsewhere that failed to disclose any tumor cells.

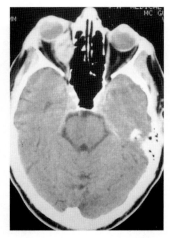

Figure 13-38. Axial computed tomography of the patient shown in Fig. 13-37 demonstrating ovoid mass in the medial aspect of the right orbit. The mass was removed.

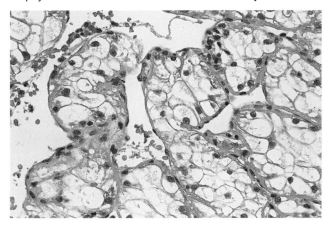

Figure 13-39. Histopathology of lesion shown in Fig. 13-37 demonstrating lobules of clear cells compatible with renal cell carcinoma (hematoxylin–eosin, original magnification × 100).

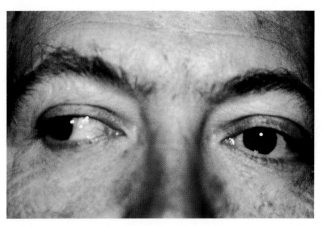

Figure 13-40. Metastatic melanoma to the medial rectus muscle. Lateral displacement of the left eye in a 43-year-old man.

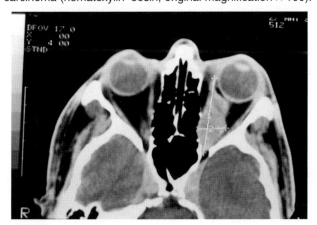

Figure 13-41. Axial computed tomography of the patient shown in Fig. 13-40 showing fusiform mass involving the medial rectus muscle.

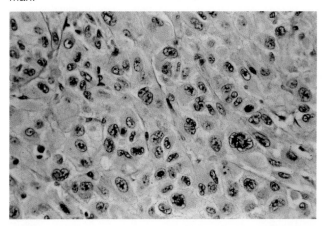

Figure 13-42. Histopathology of the lesion shown in Fig. 13-40 demonstrating malignant melanoma cells. The patient also had metastasis to axillary lymph nodes, but a primary site of the melanoma was never found (hematoxylin–eosin, original magnification × 200).

Orbital Metastasis of Neuroblastoma

In most cases of metastatic neuroblastoma, a prior diagnosis of adrenal gland neuroblastoma has been made. In exceptional cases, the orbital metastasis becomes apparent before the primary abdominal mass is found. Two such cases are illustrated.

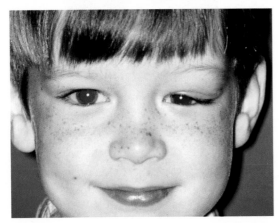

Figure 13-43. Proptosis and blepharoptosis of the left eye in a 6-year-old boy.

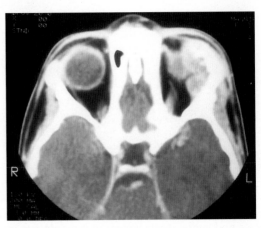

Figure 13-44. Axial computed tomography of the patient shown in 13-43 demonstrating irregular mass involving bone in superotemporal aspect of the orbit.

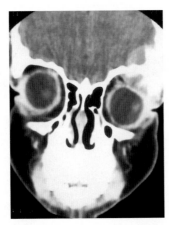

Figure 13-45. Coronal computed tomography showing the lesion depicted in Fig. 13-44. Note the extension into the cranial cavity. Biopsy revealed metastatic neuroblastoma, and the primary adrenal gland tumor was subsequently detected.

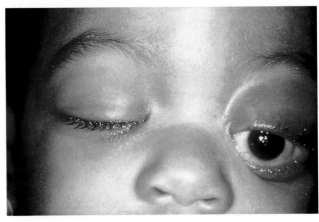

Figure 13-46. Proptosis of the left eye in a 2-year-old girl. (Courtesy of Drs. Julia Stevens and Morton Smith.)

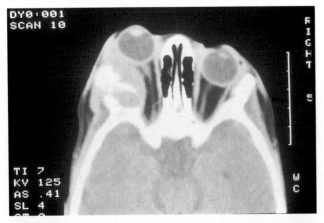

Figure 13-47. Axial computed tomography of the patient shown in Fig. 13-46 revealing a superotemporal bone destructive orbital lesion similar to the prior patient.

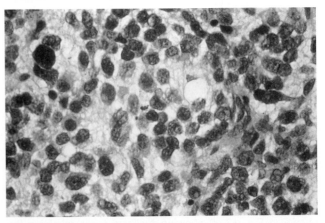

Figure 13-48. Histopathology of the lesion shown in Fig. 13-47 demonstrating malignant neuroblastic cells (hematoxylin–eosin, original magnification × 200).

Orbital Metastasis of Wilms' Tumor, Ewing's Tumor, and Rhabdomyosarcoma

Other childhood neoplasms that can metastasize to the orbit include Wilms' tumor, Ewing's tumor, and rhabdomyosarcoma.

From Shields CL, Shields JA, Mruczek AW. Enophthalmos as the initial manifestation of metastasis from scirrhous carcinoma of the breast. *Ophthalmic Pract* 1989;7:159–160.

Figs. 13-49 and 13-50 courtesy of Dr. John Purcell. From Fratkin D, Purcell JJ, Krachmer JH, et al. Wilms' tumor metastasis to the orbit. *JAMA* 1977;238:1841–1842.

Fig. 13-51 and 13-52 courtesy of Dr. Eiko Kawachi. From Kawachi E, Nunobiki K, Shimada S, et al. A case of Ewing's sarcoma with orbital metastasis. *Folia Ophthalmol Jpn* 1984;35:1840–1845.

Figs. 13-53 and 13-54 courtesy of Dr. Neil Miller. From Fekrat S, Miller NR, Loury MC. Alveolar rhabdomyosarcoma that metastasized to the orbit. *Arch Ophthalmol* 1993;111:1662–1664.

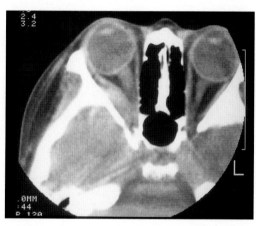

Figure 13-49. Metastatic Wilms' tumor to the right orbit.

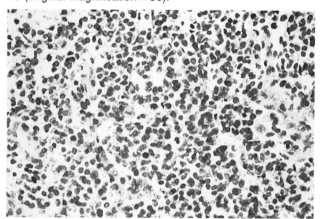

Figure 13-50. Histopathology of the lesion shown in Fig. 13-49 (original magnification × 50).

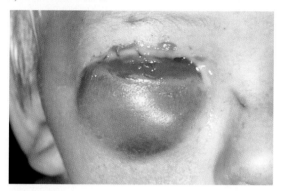

Figure 13-51. Axial computed tomography showing metastatic Ewing's sarcoma to the right orbit along the lateral rectus muscle.

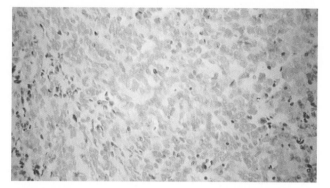

Figure 13-52. Histopathology of the lesion shown in Fig. 13-51 demonstrating small round cells characteristic of metastatic Ewing's sarcoma to the orbit.

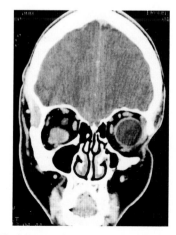

Figure 13-53. Metastatic rhabdomyosarcoma to the orbit.

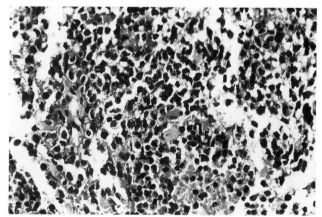

Figure 13-54. Histopathology of metastatic rhabdomyosarcoma to the orbit in a 22-year-old who had a paravaginal alveolar rhabdomyosarcoma (hematoxylin–eosin, original magnification × 100).

CHAPTER 14

Lymphoid Tumors and Leukemias

NON-HODGKIN'S B-CELL LYMPHOMA

Lymphoid tumors represent a fairly common group of orbital neoplasms. The classification and management of orbital lymphoid neoplasms is difficult and controversial, and is discussed elsewhere (1,2). To simplify, lymphoid tumors in the orbit and ocular adnexa can be benign (reactive lymphoid hyperplasia), intermediate, or malignant. It often is difficult to determine clinically whether a particular lesion is benign or malignant, and histopathologic evaluation by an experienced pathologist is necessary to accurately categorize these lesions. The term lymphoma is used here to describe all of these lesions. In general, orbital lymphoma has rather characteristic clinical, radiographic, and pathologic features. It generally occurs in older individuals but can occur in young patients who are immunosuppressed (2). Burkitt's lymphoma also can affect the orbit of children (3). Orbital lymphoma usually presents as a painless, slowly progressive, unilateral or bilateral anterior orbital mass, which may be palpable through the eyelid or conjunctiva as a rubbery mass. It is important in such cases to inspect the conjunctiva for a typical fleshy (salmon patch) infiltration and to check the uveal tract for iris or choroidal infiltration that, if present, strongly suggests that the orbital lesion is lymphoma. Computed tomography and magnetic resonance imaging disclose an ovoid or elongated mass that tends to mold to adjacent orbital structures. With histopathology and immunohistochemistry, most benign or malignant orbital lymphomas are of the B-cell type. A significant proportion of orbital and adnexal lymphoid tumors are extranodal and of the recently described mucosal-associated lymphoid tissue type (2).

Management of suspected orbital lymphoma is individualized to each case. An orbital biopsy generally is advisable, and the best approach is determined by imaging studies. Prior communication with an experienced pathologist is crucial so that the excised tissue can be processed appropriately. The surgeon should remove as much of the orbital tumor as possible without damage to the optic nerve, extraocular muscles, or other structures. In general, a physical examination and laboratory and imaging studies should be done to rule out systemic lymphoma. If systemic lymphoma is present and chemotherapy is advised, then the orbital lesion can be followed with no further treatment. If no systemic lymphoma is found, then the orbital lymphoma can be treated with radiotherapy. About 2,000 to 2,500 cGy is given for more benign lesions and about 3,500 to 4,000 cGy for malignant lesions. The patient should have continued follow-up for the development of systemic lymphoma.

SELECTED REFERENCES

1. Shields JA. *Diagnosis and management of orbital tumors.* Philadelphia: WB Saunders, 1989:291–315.
2. Cockerham GC, Jakobiec FA. Lymphoproliferative disorders of the ocular adnexa. *Int Ophthalmol Clin* 1997;37:39–59.
3. Edelstein C, Shields JA, Shields CL, De Potter P, Eagle RC Jr, Turtel L, Hagstrom N. Non-African Burkitt's lymphoma presenting with oral thrush and an orbital mass in a child. *Am J Ophthalmol* 1997;124:859–861.

Non-Hodgkin's B-cell Lymphoma—Clinical and Radiographic Features

Orbital lymphoma has characteristic clinical and radiographic features that should strongly suggest the diagnosis.

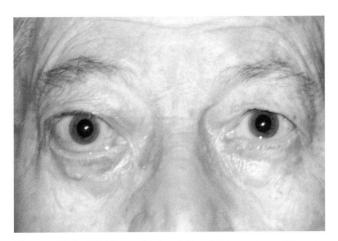

Figure 14-1. Slight proptosis of the right eye in a 90-year-old man with no prior history of lymphoma.

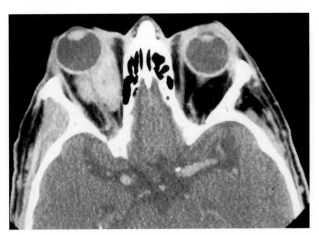

Figure 14-2. Axial computed tomography of the patient shown in Fig. 14-1. Note the characteristic diffuse orbital mass that molds to the globe and optic nerve. In such a case, incisional biopsy can be done under local anesthesia.

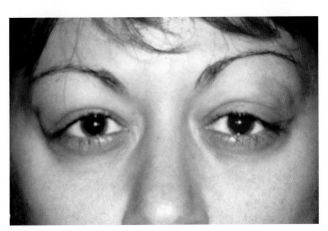

Figure 14-3. Bilateral lacrimal gland involvement by lymphoma. Note the superotemporal orbital fullness bilaterally in this 37-year-old woman.

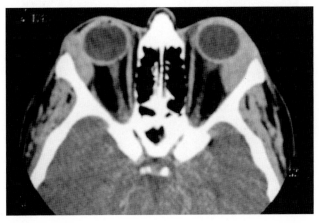

Figure 14-4. Axial computed tomography of the patient shown in Fig. 14-3 showing the bilateral orbital masses that mold to the globe and orbital bone.

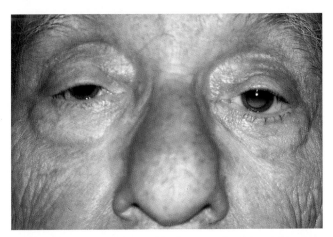

Figure 14-5. Proptosis and blepharoptosis of the right eye in an 86-year-old man.

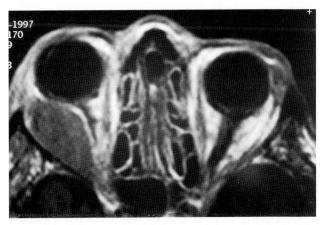

Figure 14-6. Axial magnetic resonance imaging in T1-weighted image showing a diffuse ovoid mass in temporal aspect of orbit.

Non-Hodgkin's B-cell Lymphoma—Clinical Variations and Pathology

In a patient with suspected orbital lymphoma, it is important to perform a complete ocular examination. The finding of typical lymphoma of the conjunctiva or uveal tract should strongly suggest that the orbital lesion is lymphoma. A case is illustrated.

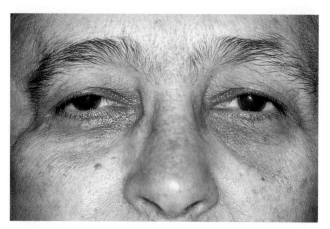

Figure 14-7. Minimal blepharoptosis and proptosis of the right eye in a 68-year-old woman.

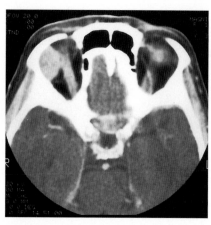

Figure 14-8. Axial computed tomography showing an ovoid mass in the superotemporal aspect of the orbit.

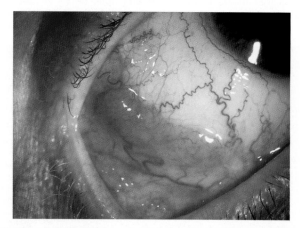

Figure 14-9. Subtle lymphoid infiltration in the inferotemporal conjunctival fornix.

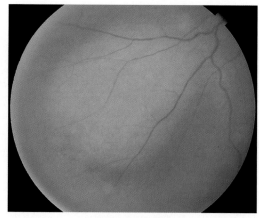

Figure 14-10. Yellow-orange lymphoid infiltrate in the choroid inferotemporally. The patient had declined treatment, and the orbital, conjunctival, and choroidal lesions enlarged very slowly.

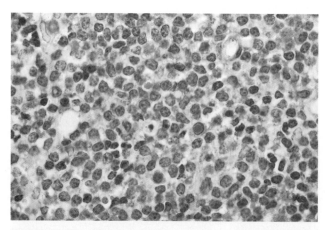

Figure 14-11. Histopathology of another case showing low-grade orbital lymphoma. Note the well-differentiated lymphocytes and the eosinophilic intranuclear inclusion body (Dutcher body) near the center of the field (hematoxylin–eosin, original magnification × 200).

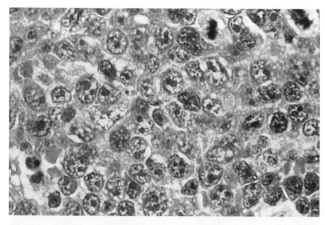

Figure 14-12. Histopathology of malignant orbital lymphoma showing poorly-differentiated lymphocytes (hematoxylin–eosin, original magnification × 200).

Non-Hodgkin's B-cell Lymphoma—Management

In most instances, a biopsy is indicated for suspected orbital lymphoma. If there is no known lymphoma, an open biopsy is done. Small anterior circumscribed tumors should be excised completely if possible. Large nonresectable tumors should have incisional biopsy, still removing as much of the tumor as possible. It the patient has known lymphoma that has already been diagnosed and staged, fine-needle aspiration biopsy can be performed to confirm the orbital diagnosis. The orbital tumor can respond to either irradiation or chemotherapy.

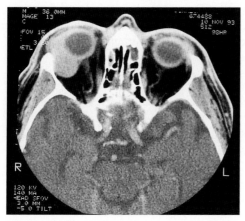

Figure 14-13. Axial computed tomography showing well-circumscribed orbital lymphoma involving the lacrimal gland. Because the tumor requires a biopsy and is surgically accessible, it is advisable to remove the tumor entirely, rather than performing an incisional biopsy.

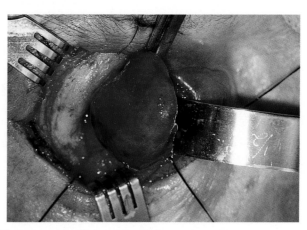

Figure 14-14. Entire tumor being removed through superotemporal orbitotomy without an osteotomy.

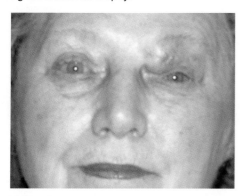

Figure 14-15. Superonasal anterior orbital mass presenting as a subcutaneous lesion in a 71-year-old woman with known lymphoma. In such a case, fine-needle aspiration biopsy performed in the office is sufficient to confirm the suspected diagnosis.

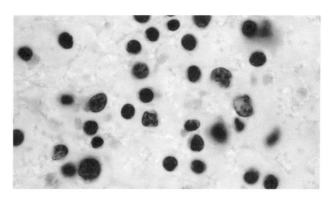

Figure 14-16. Cytology of fine-needle aspiration biopsy of the patient shown in Fig. 14-15. Note the large and small lymphocytes.

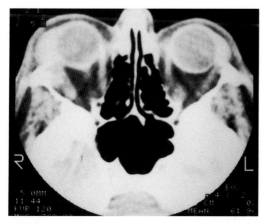

Figure 14-17. Response of orbital lymphoma to irradiation. Axial computed tomography shows a diffuse right temporal orbital mass in a 70-year-old man.

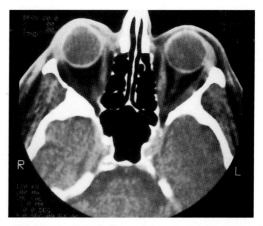

Figure 14-18. Postirradiation axial computed tomography of the patient shown in Fig. 14-17 demonstrating complete regression of the tumor.

ORBITAL LYMPHOMA—ATYPICAL FORMS

Most orbital lymphomas are typical non-Hodgkin's B-cell lymphoma (1). However, unusual variants do occur. An example of a large-cell lymphoma with microvillous projections is shown. This rare form of lymphoma may be confused with an epithelial tumor by light microscopy and even electron microscopy (2).

Cutaneous T-cell lymphoma (mycosis fungoides) also can affect the orbit (3). It appears to be much more aggressive than B-cell lymphoma and can grow rapidly and destroy the eye. Most patients already have systemic T-cell lymphoma. The treatment is similar to that described for B-cell lymphoma. The prognosis is guarded.

SELECTED REFERENCES

1. Shields JA. *Diagnosis and management of orbital tumors.* Philadelphia: WB Saunders, 1989:41–42.
2. Font RL, Shields JA. Large cell lymphoma of the orbit with microvillous projections ("porcupine lymphoma"). *Arch Ophthalmol* 1985;103:1715–1719.
3. Meekins B, Proia AD, Klintworth GK. Cutaneous T-cell lymphoma presenting as rapidly enlarging ocular adnexal tumor. *Ophthalmology* 1985;91:1288–1293.

Large-cell Lymphoma with Microvillus Projections and Cutaneous T-cell Lymphoma

Figs. 14-19 through 14-22 from Font RL, Shields JA. Large cell lymphoma of the orbit with microvillous projections ("porcupine lymphoma"). *Arch Ophthalmol* 1985;103:1715–1719.

Figs. 14-23 and 14-24 courtesy of Dr. Alan Proia. From Meekins B, Proia AD, Klintworth GK. Cutaneous T-cell lymphoma presenting as rapidly enlarging ocular adnexal tumor. *Ophthalmology* 1985;91;1288–1293.

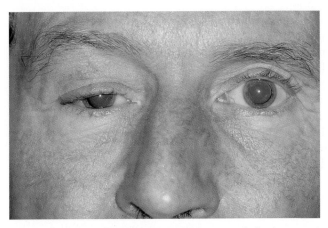

Figure 14-19. Blepharoptosis and downward displacement of the right eye in a 57-year-old man.

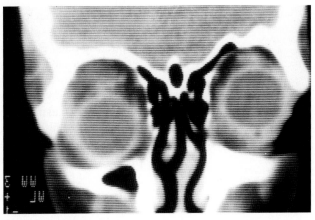

Figure 14-20. Coronal computed tomography showing a superotemporal orbital mass. There was bone erosion evident on many sections.

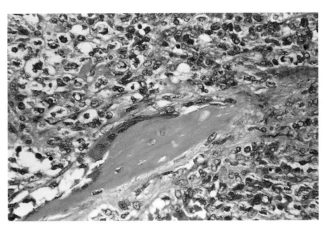

Figure 14-21. Histopathology showing anaplastic tumor cells. The diagnosis could not be determined on the basis of light microscopy (hematoxylin–eosin, original magnification × 100).

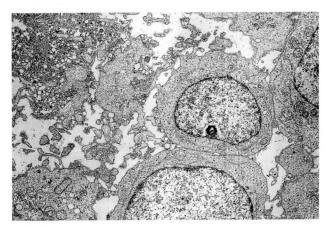

Figure 14-22. Electron photomicrograph showing lymphoid cells with microvillus projections, resembling an epithelial tumor. However, these findings are characteristic of a large-cell lymphoma with microvillus projections ("porcupine" lymphoma).

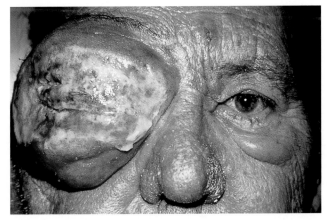

Figure 14-23. Massive orbital involvement and destruction of the eye by aggressive T-cell lymphoma (mycosis fungoides).

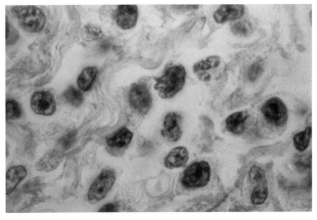

Figure 14-24. Histopathology of the lesion shown in Fig. 14-23 demonstrating malignant T-cells.

LYMPHOPLASMACYTOID AND PLASMA CELL TUMORS

Closely related to lymphoma are the lymphoplasmacytoid tumors and plasma cell tumors (1–3). Lymphoplasmacytoid tumors are composed of B-lymphocytes and plasma cells. The plasma cell is actually a B-lymphocyte that produces large amounts of immunoglobulin. The clinical and radiographic features are similar to B-cell lymphoma and the management is the same. Some patients will eventually develop multiple myeloma or related conditions.

Pure plasmacytoma can involve the orbit as a solitary lesion or as part of multiple myeloma. The solitary extramedullary plasmacytoma occurs usually in the upper respiratory tract, gastrointestinal tract, or lymph nodes and is rare in the orbit, where it can occur as a soft-tissue lesion. Management is biopsy confirmation followed by radiotherapy if the tumor is not removed completely.

Multiple myeloma is a plasma cell neoplasm characterized by plasma cell infiltration of bone marrow and by monoclonal immunoglobulin in the serum. It occasionally can affect the bone and orbital soft tissue as part of the disease process. Multiple myeloma usually is treated with radiation to local lesions, systemic chemotherapy, and bone marrow transplant. Orbital myeloma often is treated with radiation (3).

SELECTED REFERENCES

1. Shields JA. *Diagnosis and management of orbital tumors.* Philadelphia: WB Saunders, 1989:41–42.
2. Shields JA, Cooper H, Donoso LA, Augsburger JJ, Arbizo V. Immunohistochemical and ultrastructural study of unusual IgM lambda lymphoplasmacytic tumor of the lacrimal gland. *Am J Ophthalmol* 1986;101:451–457.
3. Adkins JW, Shields JA, Shields CL, Eagle RC Jr, Flanagan JC, Campanella PC. Plasmacytoma of the eye and orbit. *Int Ophthalmol* 1977;20:339–343.

Lymphoplasmacytoid and Plasma Cell Tumors

Figs. 14-25 through 14-27 from Shields JA, Cooper H, Donoso LA, Augsburger JJ, Arbizo V. Immunohistochemical and ultrastructural study of unusual IgM lambda lymphoplasmacytic tumor of the lacrimal gland. *Am J Ophthalmol* 1986;101:451–457.

Figs. 14-28 through 14-30 from Adkins JW, Shields JA, Shields CL, Eagle RC Jr, Flanagan JC, Campanella PC. Plasmacytoma of the eye and orbit. *Int Ophthalmol* 1977;20:339–343.

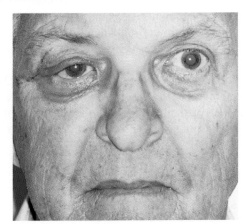

Figure 14-25. Lymphoplasmacytoid tumor. Blepharoptosis and slight proptosis of the right eye of a 72-year-old man.

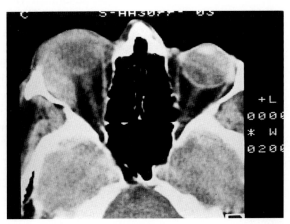

Figure 14-26. Axial computed tomography of the patient shown in Fig. 14-25 depicting an ovoid tumor in the superotemporal orbit. The tumor was completely excised via a superotemporal orbitotomy.

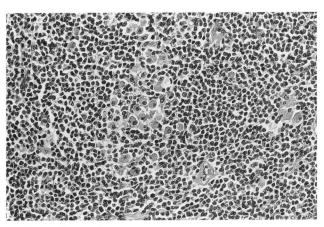

Figure 14-27. Histopathology of the lesion shown in Fig. 14-26 demonstrating diffuse sheets of small lymphocytes with foci of swollen plasma cells (hematoxylin–eosin, original magnification × 100).

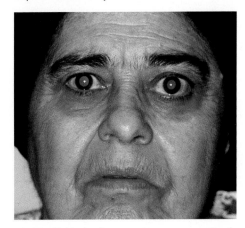

Figure 14-28. Orbital plasmacytoma as part of multiple myeloma. A 76-year-old woman with a 3-year history of IgG lambda multiple myeloma treated with chemotherapy developed proptosis of the left eye.

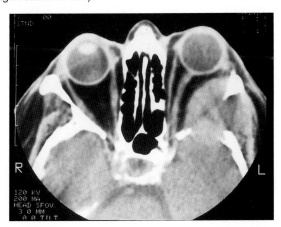

Figure 14-29. Axial computed tomography of the patient shown in Fig. 14-28 demonstrating diffuse temporal orbital mass with medial displacement of the optic nerve and destruction of the zygomatic bone.

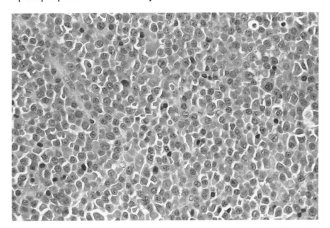

Figure 14-30. Histopathology of the lesion shown in Fig. 14-29 demonstrating sheets of atypical plasma cells (hematoxylin–eosin, original magnification × 75).

BURKITT'S LYMPHOMA

Burkitt's lymphoma was originally described as a tumor that was endemic in children from certain regions of Africa (1). It comprises approximately 50% of childhood malignant tumors in East Africa (2). It generally involved the bones of the jaws, orbit, and abdominal viscera. Subsequently, three distinct forms—the African type, non-African (American) type, and an acquired immune deficiency (AIDS) type—have been recognized, any of which can involve the orbit (3–5). Any of the forms can occur as a soft-tissue mass or can involve orbital bone. The American type can begin in the ethmoid sinus and secondarily invade the orbit.

Histopathologically, Burkitt's lymphoma is a proliferation of closely packed B-lymphocytes. Interspersed histiocytes containing phagocytosed debris impart to the tumor the so-called starry sky appearance. Management is biopsy followed by appropriate irradiation and chemotherapy (1–5). The prognosis has improved greatly in recent years.

SELECTED REFERENCES

1. Burkitt D. A sarcoma involving the jaws in African children. *Br J Surg* 1958;46:218–223.
2. Templeton AC. Orbital tumours in African children. *Br J Ophthalmol* 1971;55:254–261.
3. Shields JA. *Diagnosis and management of orbital tumors.* Philadelphia: WB Saunders, 1989:325–330.
4. Edelstein C, Shields JA, Shields CL, De Potter P, Eagle RC Jr, Turtel L, Hagstrom N. Non-African Burkitt's lymphoma presenting with oral thrush and an orbital mass in a child. *Am J Ophthalmol* 1997;124:859–861.
5. Brooks HL, Downing J, McClure JA, et al. Orbital Burkitt's lymphoma in a homosexual man with acquired immune deficiency. *Arch Ophthalmol* 1984;102:1533–1537.

Burkitt's Lymphoma

Figs. 14-32 through 14-34 from Edelstein C, Shields JA, Shields CL, De Potter P, Eagle RC Jr, Turtel L, Hagstrom N. Non-African Burkitt's lymphoma presenting with oral thrush and an orbital mass in a child. *Am J Ophthalmol* 1997;124:859–861.

Figs. 14-35 and 14-36 courtesy of Dr. H. Logan Brooks. From Brooks HL, Downing J, McClure JA, et al. Orbital Burkitt's lymphoma in a homosexual man with acquired immune deficiency. *Arch Ophthalmol* 1984;102:1533–1537.

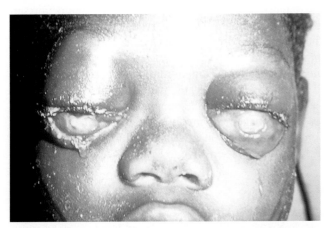

Figure 14-31. African Burkitt's lymphoma. Massive bilateral orbital involvement with secondary exposure keratopathy and corneal ulceration in an African child. (Courtesy of Armed Forces Institute of Pathology, Washington, DC.)

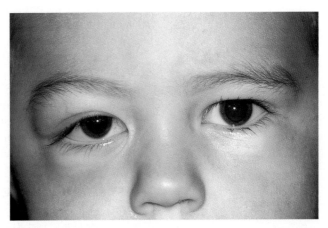

Figure 14-32. Non-African Burkitt's lymphoma. Eyelid swelling and proptosis of the right eye in a 26-month-old child.

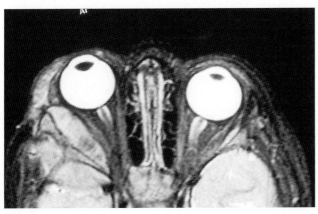

Figure 14-33. Axial magnetic resonance imaging in T2-weighted image of the patient shown in Fig. 14-32 demonstrating elongated mass along the lateral wall of the orbit.

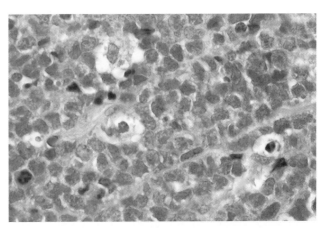

Figure 14-34. Histopathology of the lesion shown in Fig. 14-33 depicting the sheets of lymphocytes with islands of histiocytes.

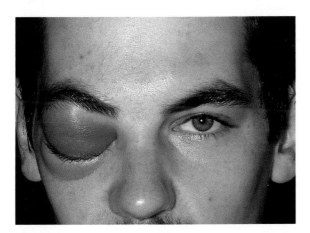

Figure 14-35. AIDS-related Burkitt's lymphoma. Acute eyelid swelling and proptosis in a teenage boy.

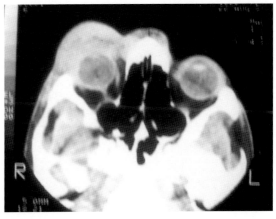

Figure 14-36. Axial computed tomography of the patient shown in Fig. 14-35 demonstrating diffuse anterior orbital involvement by the tumor. It showed a dramatic response to chemotherapy.

GRANULOCYTIC SARCOMA (LEUKEMIA)

All forms of leukemia occasionally can affect the orbit. The best known is orbital soft-tissue invasion by myelogenous leukemia, known as granulocytic sarcoma or chloroma (1–5). In one study of patients with acute myelogenous leukemia, 36% had orbital granulocytic sarcoma (3). It is well known that the orbital involvement can occur before the patient has the diagnosis of leukemia (2). Therefore, granulocytic sarcoma must be included in the differential diagnosis of otherwise healthy children with an orbital mass. Imaging studies disclose an orbital soft-tissue mass that often involves bone and extends into the temporal fossa.

Histopathologically, granulocytic sarcoma is composed of round cells that are similar to cells seen in large-cell lymphoma. However, the nuclei are more oval and the cytoplasm is more granular, a feature that can be demonstrated with the Leder stain for identification of esterase. The management involves treatment of the systemic leukemia with appropriate chemotherapeutic agents. The orbital tumor generally responds well to the chemotherapy. It also is sensitive to irradiation.

SELECTED REFERENCES

1. Shields JA. *Diagnosis and management of orbital tumors.* Philadelphia: WB Saunders, 1989:334–337.
2. Zimmerman L, Font RL. Ophthalmologic manifestations of granulocytic sarcoma (myeloid sarcoma or chloroma). *Am J Ophthalmol* 1975;30:975–990.
3. Cavdar AO, Arcasoy A, Babacan E, et al. Ocular granulocytic sarcoma (chloroma with acute myelomonocytic leukemia) in Turkish children. *Cancer* 1978;41:1606–1609.
4. Kincaid MC, Green WR. Ocular and orbital involvement in leukemia. *Surv Ophthalmol* 1983;27:211–232.
5. Michelson JB, Shields JA, Leonard BC, Caputo AR, Bergman GE. Periorbital chloroma and proptosis in a two-year old with acute myelogenous leukemia. *J Pediatr Ophthalmol* 1975;12:255–258.

Granulocytic Sarcoma (Leukemia)

Figs. 14-37 through 14-40 courtesy of Dr. Ramon Font. From Davis JL, Parke DW II, Font RL. Granulocytic sarcoma of the orbit. A clinicopathologic study. *Ophthalmology* 1985;92:1758–1762.

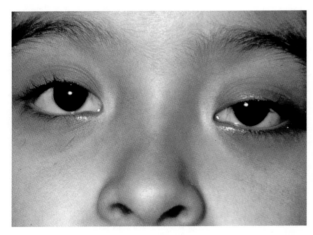

Figure 14-37. Blepharoptosis and proptosis of the left eye due to granulocytic sarcoma in a 9-year-old girl.

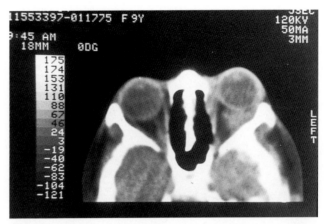

Figure 14-38. Axial computed tomography of the patient shown in Fig. 14-37 depicting an ill-defined orbital mass. Biopsy of an associated brain lesion revealed granulocytic sarcoma. It was almost 1 month later that patient developed positive results on blood studies for leukemia.

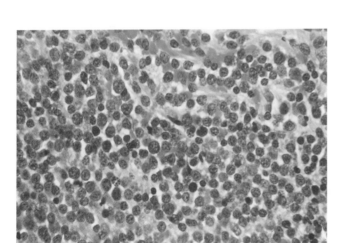

Figure 14-39. Histopathology of the tumor shown in Fig. 14-38 showing poorly differentiated blast cells (hematoxylin–eosin, original magnification × 100).

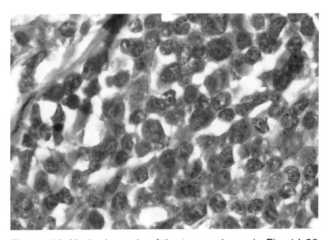

Figure 14-40. Leder stain of the tumor shown in Fig. 14-39 depicting the cytoplasmic granules (Leder, original magnification × 250).

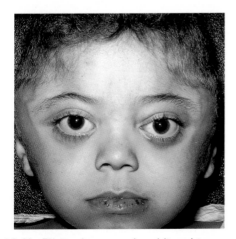

Figure 14-41. Bilateral masses in orbit and temporal fossa in a child with leukemia. Note the pallor of the skin.

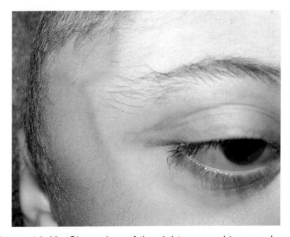

Figure 14-42. Close view of the right eye and temporal area in the child shown in Fig. 14-41. Note the dilated temporal vein.

CHAPTER 15

Secondary Orbital Tumors

SECONDARY ORBITAL TUMORS

By traditional definition, a secondary orbital tumor is one that has invaded the orbital tissues from a neoplastic site in adjacent structures, such as eyelid, conjunctiva intraocular structures, sinuses, nasopharynx, and brain (1,2).

The main eyelid tumors that can involve the orbit secondarily include basal cell carcinoma, sebaceous gland carcinoma, squamous cell carcinoma, cutaneous melanoma, and Merkel cell carcinoma (3,4). Conjunctival tumors include squamous cell carcinoma, particularly the mucoepidermoid variant, and melanoma. Wide surgical excision using a "no touch" technique is important in preventing tumor recurrence and orbital invasion (5). Intraocular tumors include uveal melanoma and retinoblastoma and, rarely, medulloepithelioma and epithelial tumors of the ciliary body (6–8). Sinus tumors that can secondarily involve the orbit include carcinoma of the ethmoid or maxillary sinus and, rarely, rhabdomyosarcoma (9). Nasopharyngeal tumors include carcinoma, juvenile angiofibroma, and esthesioneuroblastoma (10,11). Intracranial tumors include sphenoid wing meningioma and, rarely, glioblastoma. In the case of primary tumors without systemic involvement, orbital exenteration may be the best treatment (12). Most of the tumors that can secondarily invade the orbit have been discussed in other chapters and in the other atlases. A few examples of secondary orbital involvement by these neoplasms are cited here.

SELECTED REFERENCES

1. Shields JA. *Diagnosis and management of orbital tumors.* Philadelphia: WB Saunders, 1989:341–377.
2. Glover AT, Grove AS Jr. Orbital invasion by malignant eyelid tumors. *Ophthal Plast Reconstr Surg* 1989;5: 1–12.
3. Shields JA, Font RL. Meibomian gland carcinoma presenting as a lacrimal gland tumor. *Arch Ophthalmol* 1974;92:304–308.
4. Shields JA, Elder D, Arbizo V, Hedges T, Augsburger JJ. Orbital involvement with desmoplastic melanoma. *Br J Ophthalmol* 1987;71:279–285.
5. Shields JA, Shields CL, De Potter P. Surgical approach to conjunctival tumors. The 1994 Lynn B. McMahan Lecture. *Arch Ophthalmol* 1997;115:808–815.
6. Shields JA, Shields CL. Massive orbital extension of posterior uveal melanoma. *J Ophthal Plast Reconstr Surg* 1991;7:238–251.
7. Ellsworth RM. Orbital retinoblastoma. *Trans Am Ophthalmol Soc* 1974;72:79–88.
8. Shields CL, Shields JA, Baez K, Cater J, De Potter P. Optic nerve invasion of retinoblastoma. Metastatic potential and clinical risk factors. *Cancer* 1994;73:692–698.
9. Johnson LN, Krohel GB, Yeon EB, Parnes SM. Sinus tumors invading the orbit. *Ophthalmology* 1984;91: 209–217.
10. Bonovolonta G, Villari G, de Rosa G, et al. Ocular complications of juvenile angiofibroma. *Ophthalmologica* 1980;181:334–339.
11. Rakes SM, Yeatts RP, Campbell RJ. Ophthalmic manifestations of esthesioneuroblastoma. *Ophthalmology* 1985;92:1749–1753.
12. Shields JA, Shields CL, Suvarnamani C, Tantasira M, Shah P. Orbital exenteration with eyelid sparing: indications, technique and results. *Ophthalmic Surg* 1991;22:292–297.

Orbital Invasion by Eyelid Basal Cell Carcinoma

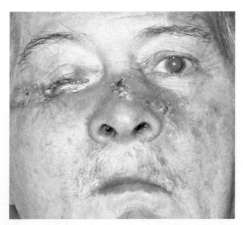

Figure 15-1. Neglected basal cell carcinoma near the lateral canthus with secondary orbital invasion in a 63-year-old man. The motility of the eye was markedly restricted due to diffuse orbital involvement.

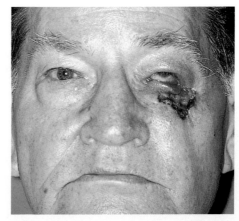

Figure 15-2. Neglected basal cell carcinoma of the lower eyelid and lateral canthus with secondary orbital invasion in a 69-year-old man. The motility of the eye was also markedly restricted.

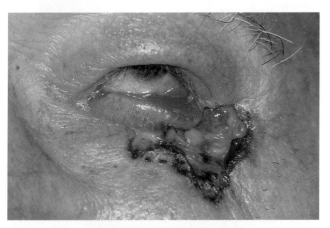

Figure 15-3. Closer view of the lesion shown in Fig. 15-2. The fibrosis in the tumor was producing a secondary ectropion of the lower eyelid.

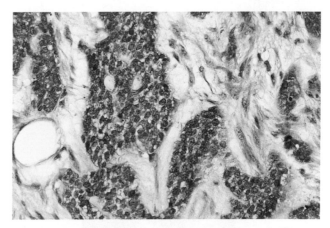

Figure 15-4. Histopathology of the lesion shown in Fig. 15-3 after orbital exenteration. Note the morpheaform basal cell carcinoma in a fibrous connective tissue stroma.

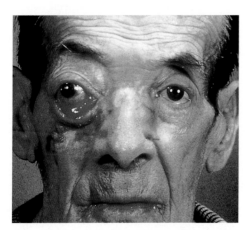

Figure 15-5. Orbital invasion by basal cell carcinoma of the lower eyelid in a 66-year-old man. He had excision of a basal cell carcinoma from right lower eyelid 16 years earlier, but he did not return for follow-up. Note that the globe is displaced superiorly and laterally. (Courtesy of Dr. Moshe Lahav.)

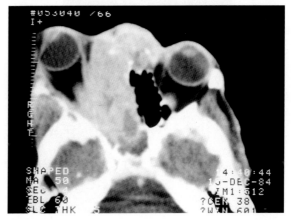

Figure 15-6. Axial computed tomography of the patient shown in Fig. 15-5. Note the massive tumor replacing the medial aspect of the orbit and ethmoid sinus with extension into the cranial cavity. (Courtesy of Dr. Moshe Lahav.)

Orbital Invasion by Sebaceous Gland Carcinoma Simulating a Primary Lacrimal Gland Tumor

Sebaceous gland carcinoma occasionally can invade the lacrimal gland tissues from a diffuse tumor in the eyelid, simulating a primary neoplasm of the lacrimal gland. A clinicopathologic correlation of such a case is shown.

From Shields JA, Font RL. Meibomian gland carcinoma presenting as a lacrimal gland tumor. *Arch Ophthalmol* 1974;92:304–308.

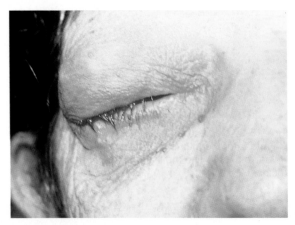

Figure 15-7. Mass in the superotemporal orbit with thickening of the upper eyelid in a 65-year-old woman.

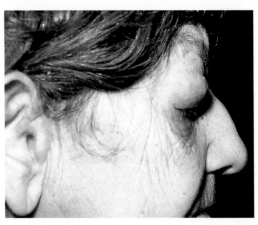

Figure 15-8. Side view showing superotemporal mass. A biopsy in the superotemporal orbit disclosed sebaceous gland carcinoma. Orbital exenteration was performed.

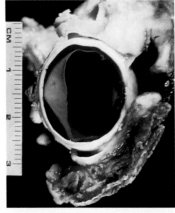

Figure 15-9. Gross exenteration specimen showing white tumor in lacrimal gland area, superior to the globe.

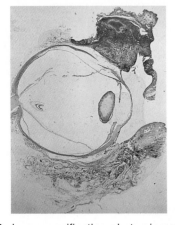

Figure 15-10. Low-magnification photomicrograph showing basophilic mass superior to the globe.

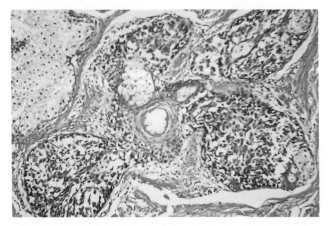

Figure 15-11. Photomicrograph of tarsal region showing lobules of sebaceous gland carcinoma (hematoxylin–eosin, original magnification × 125).

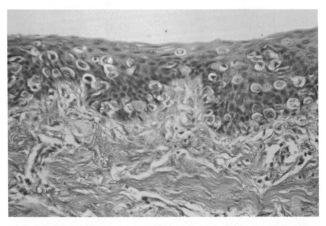

Figure 15-12. Photomicrograph showing pagetoid invasion of sebaceous gland carcinoma in the epidermis (hematoxylin–eosin, original magnification × 50).

Orbital Invasion by Eyelid Melanoma

Cutaneous melanoma has a tendency in some cases to invade the dermis by neurotropic mechanisms and to recur as a deep nodule. An eyelid melanoma can invade the soft tissues of the orbit by a similar mechanism. A case of orbital recurrence of neurotropic desmoplastic melanoma is shown.

From Shields JA, Elder D, Arbizo V, Hedges T, Augsburger JJ. Orbital involvement with desmoplastic melanoma. *Br J Ophthalmol* 1987;71:279–285.

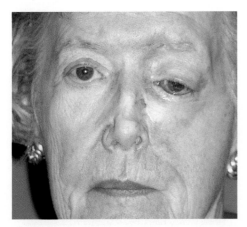

Figure 15-13. Blepharoptosis and proptosis in a 79-year-old woman who had excision of a cutaneous melanoma from the left medial canthal area 5 years earlier.

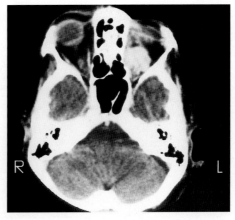

Figure 15-14. Axial computed tomography showing circumscribed tumor in the posterior aspect of the orbit.

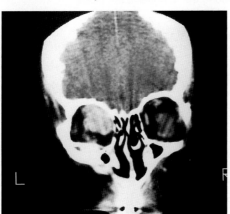

Figure 15-15. Coronal computed tomography better demonstrating the mass superiorly in the orbit.

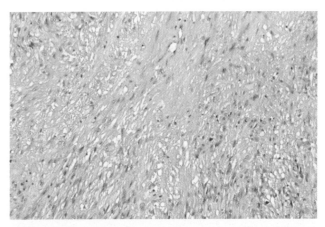

Figure 15-16. Histopathology of the lesion shown in Fig. 15-15 demonstrating marked desmoplasia with scant cells. The diagnosis of fibrous histiocytoma was initially considered (hematoxylin–eosin, original magnification × 25).

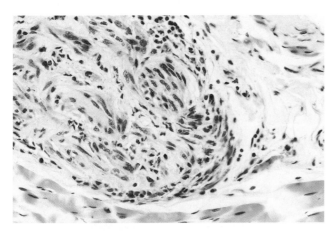

Figure 15-17. Histopathology of reexamined cutaneous lesions showing spindle cells invading a nerve (hematoxylin–eosin, original magnification × 100).

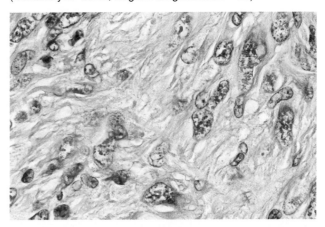

Figure 15-18. Photomicrograph of another area of orbital tumor showing anaplastic spindle and epithelioid cells. Immunohistochemistry of the original eyelid lesion and the orbital recurrence confirmed the diagnosis of melanoma (hematoxylin–eosin, original magnification × 200).

Orbital Invasion by Conjunctival Squamous Cell Carcinoma

In most instances, conjunctival squamous cell carcinoma can be controlled by carefully performed early surgery. If it is not treated early or if it is incompletely excised, orbital recurrence can develop. In such instances, eyelid-sparing orbital exenteration is often required to achieve tumor control.

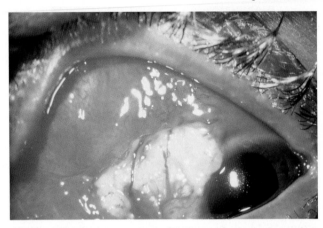

Figure 15-19. Advanced, neglected squamous cell carcinoma on the left eye of a 70-year-old man. Orbital computed tomography showed extension into the orbit with compression of the equator of the globe.

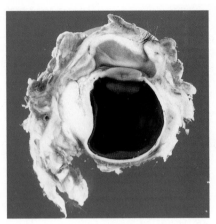

Figure 15-20. Exenteration specimen of the patient shown in Fig. 15-19 demonstrating white solid tumor extending posteriorly along the surface of the globe.

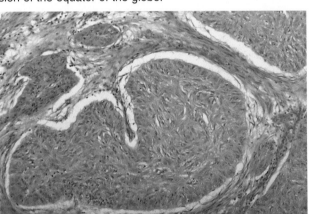

Figure 15-21. Histopathology of the lesion shown in Fig. 15-20 revealing invasive spindle-shaped spindle cells (hematoxylin–eosin, original magnification × 25).

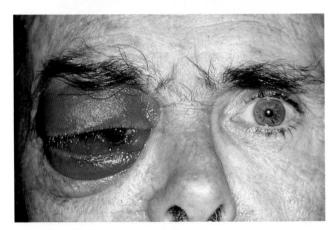

Figure 15-22. Proptosis, eyelid ecchymosis, and conjunctival hemorrhagic chemosis in a 56-year-old man who was immunosuppressed after liver transplantation. Surgery had been done elsewhere for conjunctival squamous cell carcinoma, and this represented recurrence.

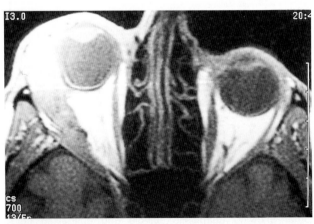

Figure 15-23. Orbital magnetic resonance imaging in T1-weighted image of the patient shown in Fig. 15-22 demonstrating tumor invasion along the lateral wall of the orbit.

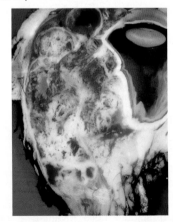

Figure 15-24. Sectioned orbital exenteration specimen demonstrating a large hemorrhagic mass temporal to the globe.

Orbital Invasion by Conjunctival Melanoma

In rare instances, conjunctival melanoma is far advanced at the time of the initial diagnosis and primary orbital exenteration is necessary. Much more commonly, however, orbital invasion of conjunctival melanoma occurs after a number of prior resections of very aggressive conjunctival melanoma. Three such cases are briefly illustrated.

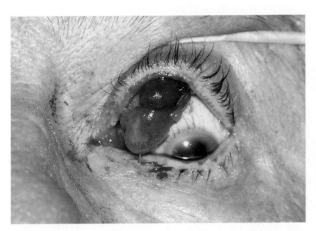

Figure 15-25. Recurrent conjunctival melanoma in the superonasal fornix with anterior orbital invasion in a 64-year-old man.

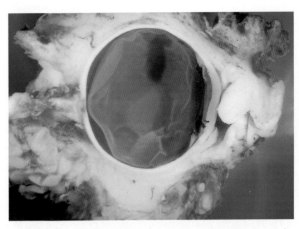

Figure 15-26. Sectioned orbital exenteration specimen from the patient shown in Fig. 15-25 revealing nodules of amelanotic melanoma anteriorly.

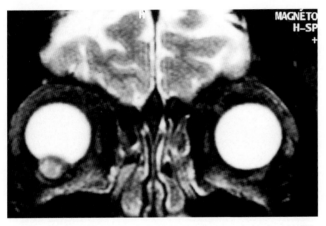

Figure 15-27. Coronal magnetic resonance imaging in T2-weighted image showing inferior orbital melanoma in a 50-year-old woman who had prior excisions of conjunctival melanoma.

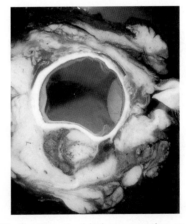

Figure 15-28. Sectioned orbital exenteration specimen from the patient shown in Fig. 15-27. Note the large tumor nodule indenting the sclera inferiorly.

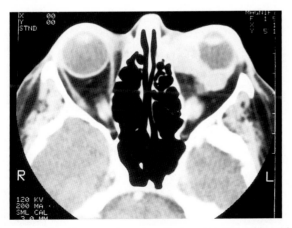

Figure 15-29. Recurrent conjunctival melanoma with orbital invasion surrounding the globe in a 72-year-old woman.

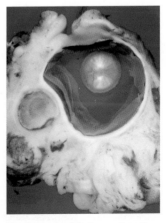

Figure 15-30. Sectioned orbital exenteration specimen from the patient shown in Fig. 15-29. Note the large tumor nodule indenting the sclera nasally.

Massive Orbital Invasion by Uveal Melanoma

On occasion, uveal melanoma can show extensive orbital invasion. It usually occurs after a long delay in diagnosis. This subject is also discussed in the *Atlas of Intraocular Tumors*. Two additional cases are illustrated here.

Figs. 15-31 through 15-33 from Shields CL, Shields JA, Yarian DL, Augsburger JJ. Intracranial extension of choroidal melanoma via the optic nerve. *Br J Ophthalmol* 1987;71:172–176.

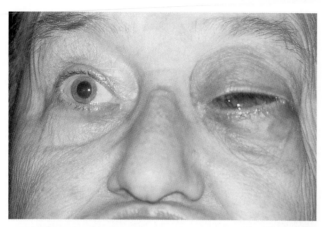

Figure 15-31. Facial view showing proptosis of the right eye in 62-year-old woman who had been treated with medication and cyclocryotherapy for "glaucoma secondary to central retinal vein occlusion" and eventually developed proptosis and pain.

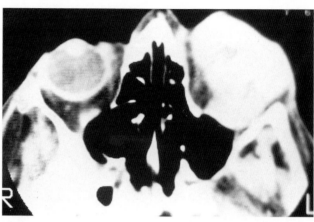

Figure 15-32. Axial computed tomography of the patient shown in Fig. 15-31 showing that the globe and the entire orbit is filled with solid tumor. A fine-needle aspiration biopsy through the inferior conjunctival fornix disclosed melanoma cells.

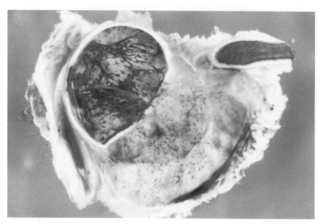

Figure 15-33. Sagittal section through the exenteration specimen of the patient shown in Fig. 15-31 showing melanoma entirely filling the globe and orbit and replacing the optic nerve.

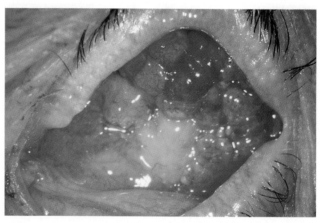

Figure 15-34. Diffuse, multinodular amelanotic epibulbar mass in a woman who underwent cataract surgery about 1 year earlier because of "phakolytic glaucoma."

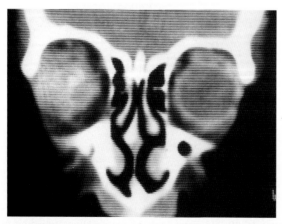

Figure 15-35. Coronal computed tomography of the patient shown in Fig. 15-33 demonstrating diffuse solid tumor encircling the globe.

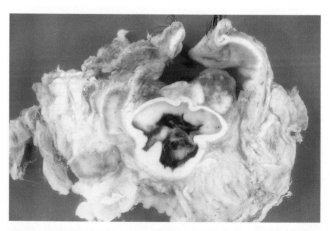

Figure 15-36. Exenteration specimen showing diffuse amelanotic ciliary body melanoma with massive extension outside the globe.

Orbital Invasion by Retinoblastoma

Retinoblastoma occasionally can exhibit extensive orbital invasion. This is rare in medically developed countries, but it is fairly common in areas of the world where advanced medical care may not be readily available. Orbital extensions of retinoblastoma generally is associated with a worse prognosis. This subject is discussed in the *Atlas of Intraocular Tumors*. Four examples are cited here.

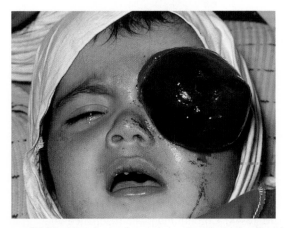

Figure 15-37. Massive extraocular extension of retinoblastoma in a child from Iran. (Courtesy of Dr. Hormoz Chams.)

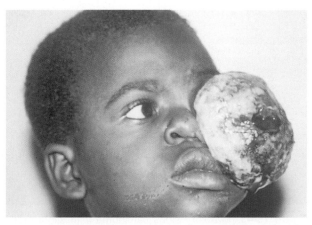

Figure 15-38. Massive extraocular extension of retinoblastoma in a child from Nigeria. (Courtesy of Dr. R. Connor and Armed Forces Institute of Pathology, Washington, DC.)

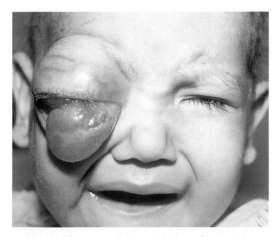

Figure 15-39. Marked orbital extension of retinoblastoma in a child from Venezuela. (Courtesy of Dr. Imelda Pifano.)

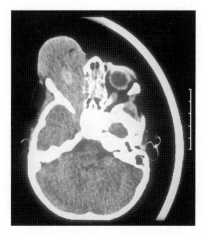

Figure 15-40. Axial computed tomography of the patient shown in Fig. 15-39 demonstrating massive intraocular and orbital tumor.

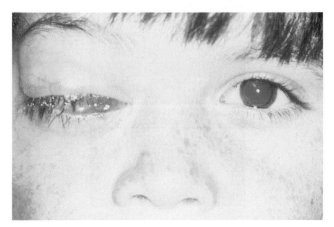

Figure 15-41. Extensive orbital swelling in a 10-year-old boy who had undergone prior enucleation elsewhere for retinoblastoma.

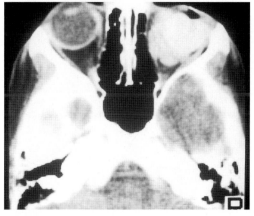

Figure 15-42. Axial computed tomography of the patient shown in Fig. 15-41 demonstrating massive retinoblastoma surrounding the orbital implant.

Orbital Extension from Paranasal Sinus Tumors

Orbital extension can develop from sinus cancers, particularly those that arise in the ethmoid or maxillary sinus. Although the majority are squamous neoplasms, a variety of sarcomas, osseous, and fibroosseous tumors can originate in the sinuses and secondarily invade the orbit. As expected, ethmoid sinus carcinoma tends to displace the globe laterally and maxillary sinus carcinoma displaces the globe superiorly. Treatment of squamous carcinoma with orbital invasion involves surgical excision in conjunction with an otolaryngologist with appropriate irradiation and chemotherapy.

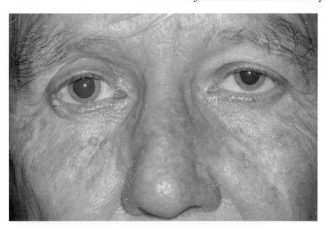

Figure 15-43. Maxillary sinus carcinoma with slight orbital extension. Slight upward displacement of the left eye in a 68-year-old man.

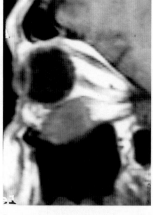

Figure 15-44. Coronal magnetic resonance imaging in T1-weighted image of the patient shown in Fig. 15-43 demonstrating a mass arising from the roof of the maxillary sinus with preferential growth into the orbital soft tissues.

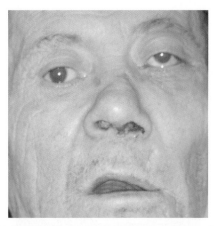

Figure 15-45. Maxillary sinus carcinoma with marked orbital extension. Upward displacement of the left eye in an 80-year-old man.

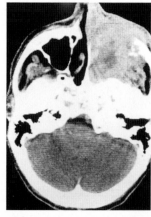

Figure 15-46. Axial computed tomography of the patient shown in Fig. 15-45 depicting massive neoplasm in the maxillary sinus.

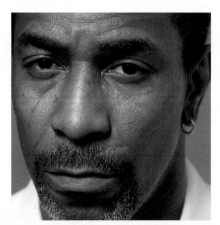

Figure 15-47. Ethmoid sinus carcinoma with orbital extension. Slight lateral displacement of the left eye in a 46-year-old man.

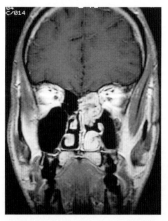

Figure 15-48. Coronal magnetic resonance imaging of the patient shown in Fig. 15-47. Note the mass in the ethmoid sinus and nasal cavity with extension into the medial aspect of the orbit.

Orbital Extension from Nasopharyngeal Tumors

Nasopharyngeal neoplasms can also secondarily invade the orbit. Nasopharyngeal carcinoma is most common but a number of other tumors can exhibit similar behavior. Tumors in this location can produce involvement of multiple cranial nerves. Juvenile angiofibroma is an uncommon tumor that affects young males. It is locally invasive, but does not tend to metastasize. Esthesioneuroblastoma is a neurogenic neoplasm that arises from the olfactory sensory epithelium in the roof of the nasal cavity.

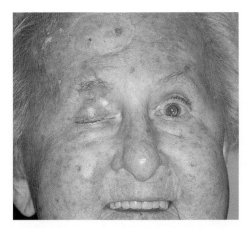

Figure 15-49. Blepharoptosis and ophthalmoplegia in an 84-year-old woman with nasopharyngeal carcinoma.

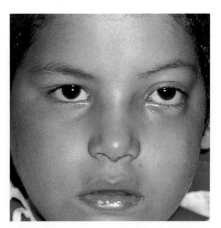

Figure 15-50. Nasopharyngeal angiofibroma. Proptosis and upward displacement of the left eye in a 7-year-old girl. A large vascular mass subsequently was removed. (Courtesy of Dr. Robert Levine.)

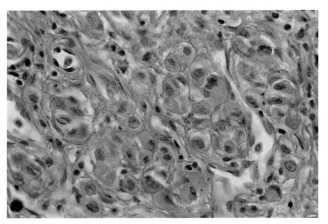

Figure 15-51. Histopathology of the mass removed from the patient shown in Fig. 15-50 demonstrating vascular neoplasm with ovoid and spindle cells (hematoxylin–eosin, original magnification × 150). (Courtesy of Dr. Robert Levine.)

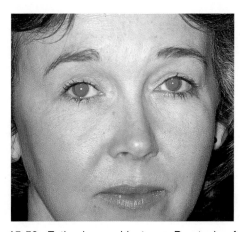

Figure 15-52. Esthesioneuroblastoma. Proptosis of the left eye in a 39-year-old woman.

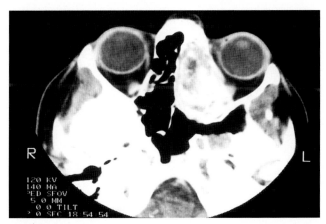

Figure 15-53. Axial computed tomography of the patient shown in Fig. 15-52 demonstrating a large irregular mass involving the nasal cavity and medial aspect of the orbit.

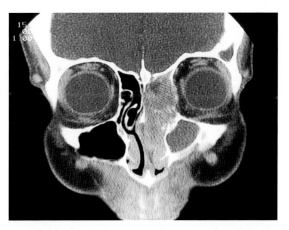

Figure 15-54. Coronal computed tomography of the lesion shown in Fig. 15-53.

CHAPTER 16

Surgical Approaches to Orbital Tumors

SURGICAL METHODS FOR ORBITAL TUMORS

The details of surgical approaches to orbital tumors and pseudotumors are discussed elsewhere (1,2). Illustrated and briefly described here are the indications and techniques of orbital fine-needle aspiration biopsy, conjunctival approach, cutaneous approaches, and orbital exenteration.

Fine-needle aspiration biopsy is a useful method for obtaining a diagnosis in selected cases (1,3). It is used most often to confirm the diagnosis of orbital lymphoma or metastasis in a patient who has known systemic lymphoma or a primary neoplasm. If lymphoma or metastasis is suspected and there is no known systemic malignancy, incisional or excisional biopsy usually should be done in order to provide more tissue for histopathologic study. Fine-needle aspiration biopsy should not be used for circumscribed orbital tumors in which complete excision is anticipated. Cases in which fine-needle aspiration biopsy is indicated have been illustrated throughout this atlas.

In general, well-circumscribed tumors should be managed with excisional biopsy, and poorly circumscribed diffuse tumors are best managed by incisional biopsy. A conjunctival approach is frequently best for selected anterior orbital tumors. It usually requires less surgical time and avoids performing a skin incision and suture removal. The authors use it more frequently for circumscribed anterior orbital tumors that are most likely benign, such as cavernous hemangioma, neurilemoma, soft-tissue dermoid cysts, and other circumscribed tumors. Circumscribed tumors in the lacrimal gland fossa, where malignancies such as adenoid cystic carcinoma are possible, generally should not be removed by a conjunctival approach. A superotemporal cutaneous incision with an extraperiosteal approach is preferable in such cases, because it allows better exposure and wider tumor removal with less chance of capsular rupture.

Cutaneous approaches are used for larger, more posteriorly located tumors and for tumors of the lacrimal gland fossa. Depending on the location and size of the lesion as determined by axial and coronal imaging studies, the incision should be made superotemporally, superonasally, inferotemporally, inferonasally, or directly nasally. Either a transeptal or transperiosteal entry into the orbit can be used, also depending on the imaging and surgical findings. Blunt dissection should be employed much as possible in the orbital soft tissues.

Orbital exenteration is used for massive orbital extension of uveal melanoma, for orbital extension of primary eyelid and conjunctival malignancies, and for certain primary orbital malignancies. When possible, an eyelid-sparing technique should be employed (4).

SELECTED REFERENCES

1. Shields JA. *Diagnosis and management of orbital tumors.* Philadelphia: WB Saunders, 1989:47–66.
2. Rootman J, Stewart B, Goldberg RA. *Orbital surgery. A conceptual approach.* Philadelphia: Lippincott–Raven Publishers, 1995.
3. Kennerdell JS, Dekker A, Johnson BL, et al. Fine needle aspiration biopsy. Its use in orbital tumors. *Arch Ophthalmol* 1979;97:1315–1317.
4. Shields JA, Shields CL, Suvarnamani C, Tantasira M, Shah P. Orbital exenteration with eyelid sparing: indications, technique and results. *Ophthalmic Surg* 1991;22:292–297.

Orbital Surgery Instrumentation and Conjunctival Approach

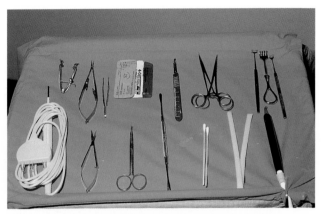

Figure 16-1. Aspiration instrument used for fine-needle aspiration biopsy of orbital tumors.

Figure 16-2. Instrument tray for orbital surgery.

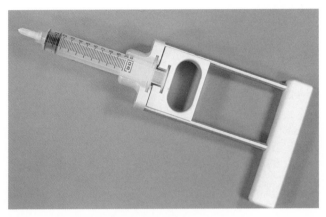

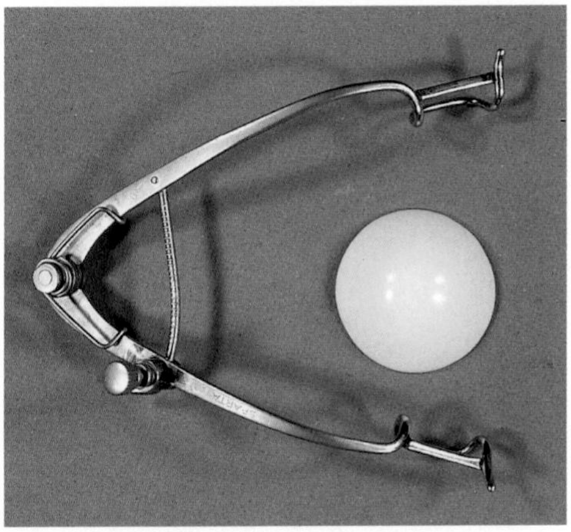

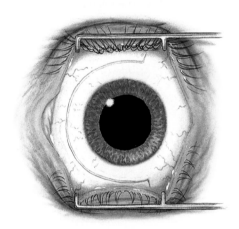

Figure 16-3. Eyelid speculum and corneal shield used for orbital surgery.

Figure 16-4. Conjunctival incision for removal of medial orbital tumor.

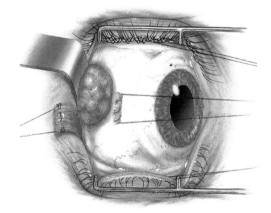

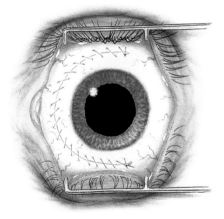

Figure 16-5. Tumor exposed after incision through conjunctiva and Tenon's capsule. Note that, in this case, the medial rectus muscle was disinserted for better exposure. In most cases, it is not necessary to disinsert the muscle.

Figure 16-6. Closure with running absorbable suture after tumor removal.

Cutaneous Superonasal Approach

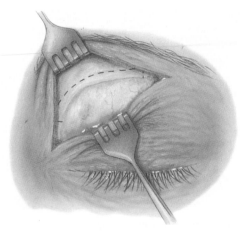

Figure 16-7. The skin incision has been made and dissection carried through the orbicularis muscle to expose the periosteum. *Dotted line* indicates where the periosteum is to be cut.

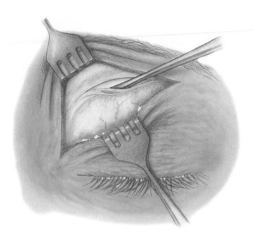

Figure 16-8. The periosteum has been incised and a periosteal elevator is being used to separate the periosteum from the orbital wall, exposing the bone.

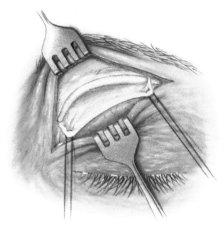

Figure 16-9. The periorbitum is exposed and ready for incision to enter the orbit.

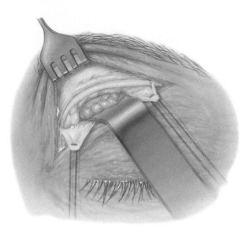

Figure 16-10. The periorbitum has been incised and soft-tissue dissection has revealed the tumor to be removed.

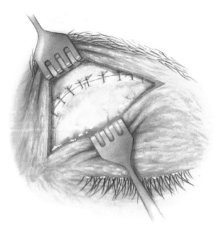

Figure 16-11. The tumor has been removed and the periosteum is closed with interrupted 5-0 absorbable sutures.

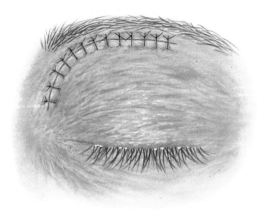

Figure 16-12. The skin has been closed with interrupted 6-0 silk sutures.

Cutaneous Superotemporal Approach

For more accessible tumors, the tumor can be removed by this approach without performing an osteotomy.

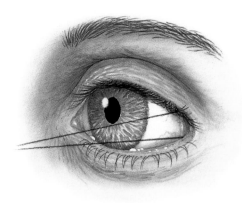

Figure 16-13. A traction suture is first placed beneath the lateral rectus muscle for traction and for identification of the muscle during surgery.

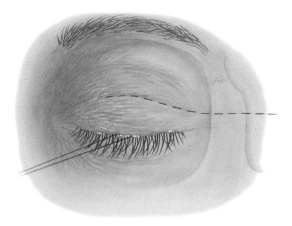

Figure 16-14. *Dotted line* indicates the location of the eyelid crease incision for superolateral orbitotomy.

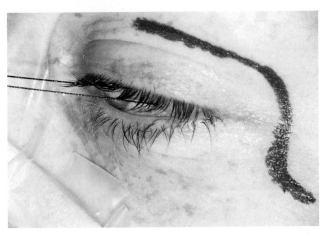

Figure 16-15. Marking pen has been used to outline the incision of a superolateral orbitotomy.

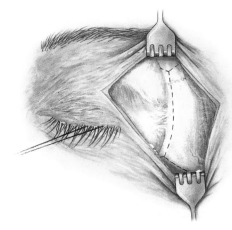

Figure 16-16. Outline of periosteal incisions shown by *dotted lines*.

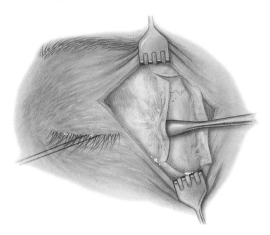

Figure 16-17. The skin, orbicularis muscle, and periosteum have been incised and a periosteal elevator is being used to separate the periosteum from the bone as was shown for the medial approach in Fig. 16-8.

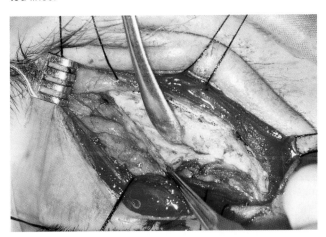

Figure 16-18. Photograph of periosteal elevator in use. When the periorbitum has been separated from the bone, a decision must be made as to whether to incise the periorbitum and remove the tumor or to perform an osteotomy (Kronlein) for better exposure.

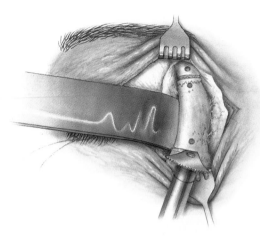

Figure 16-19. A decision has been made to perform an osteotomy. Four holes are drilled through the bone for reconstruction later and two cuts with an electrical saw are made through the bone between the holes.

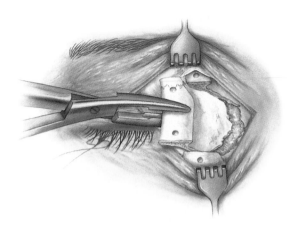

Figure 16-20. The bone flap is broken and reflected with a bone rongeur.

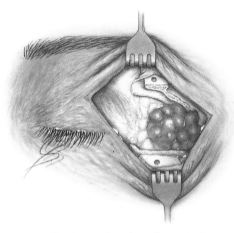

Figure 16-21. The bone flap is reflected, the periorbitum incised, and soft-tissue dissection has allowed exposure of the tumor.

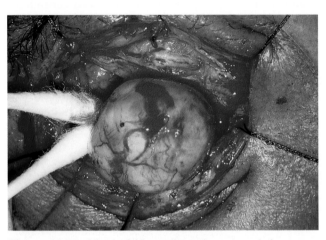

Figure 16-22. View of blunt dissection around the tumor with cotton-tipped applicators. The periosteal elevator also can be used to create a separation between the tumor and the adjacent soft tissue.

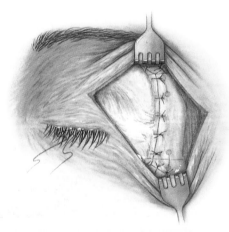

Figure 16-23. The tumor has been removed, the bone flap replaced with sutures through the drill holes, and the periosteum has been sutured.

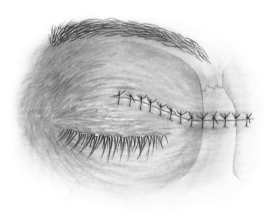

Figure 16-24. The skin has been closed with interrupted 6-0 silk sutures.

Orbital Exenteration

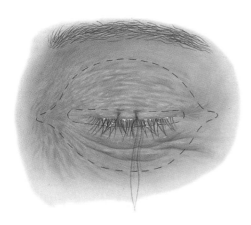

Figure 16-25. It is important to decide whether to remove the eyelids with the specimen or to spare the eyelid. The *outer dotted line* shows the incision for removing the eyelids and the *inner dotted line*, just outside the cilia, shows the incision for an eyelid-sparing technique.

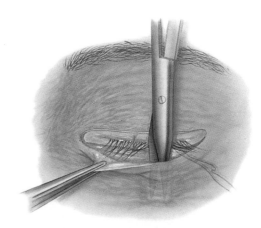

Figure 16-26. The skin incision has been made for an eyelid-sparing exenteration and the skin is separated for 360 degrees to the periosteum around the orbital rim.

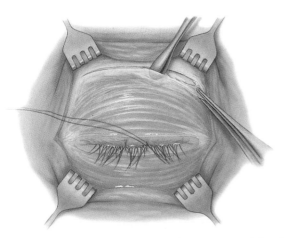

Figure 16-27. The periosteum has been exposed for 360 degrees and is being separated from the bone with a periosteal elevator.

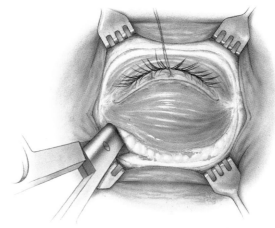

Figure 16-28. After the periorbitum is separated from bone almost to the orbital apex, long scissors are inserted between the bone and the periorbitum and used to cut the optic nerve, allowing removal of the orbital contents mostly within the periorbitum.

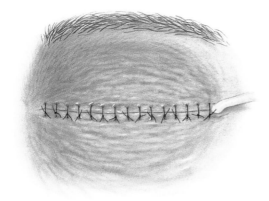

Figure 16-29. After hemostasis is achieved at the orbital apex, the eyelid flaps are sutured together and a drain is inserted.

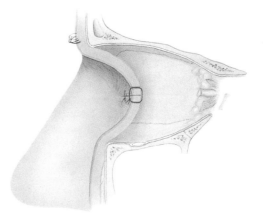

Figure 16-30. Side view showing eyelids sutured together with interrupted 5-0 nonabsorbable sutures.

Subject Index

Figures are noted with a page number followed
by the notation for the specific figure in italic
numerals: for example, figure 1-27 on page 9 is
shown as 9:*1-27*.